EAT TO BEAT EPI

Exocrine Pancreatic Insufficiency Diet Plan, Recipes, Complementary Therapies, Lifestyle Modifications For Holistic Management, And More

DR. LONDYN DELANEY

Copyright © 2024 By Dr. Londyn Delaney

All Rights Reserved...

Table of Contents

Introductory 5

CHAPTER ONE 9

   What Is Exocrine Pancreatic Insufficiency (EPI) 9

CHAPTER TWO 22

   Introduction To Enzyme Replacement Therapy (ERT) 22

   Types Of Enzymes 30

   Dosage And Administration 37

CHAPTER THREE 46

   Combining ERT With The EPI Diet 46

   Meal Planning And Preparation 55

CHAPTER FOUR 63

   Breakfast Recipes 63

CHAPTER FIVE 101

   Lunch Recipes 101

CHAPTER SIX 134

   Dinner Recipes 134

CHAPTER SEVEN 167

Snack And Dessert Recipes.................167

CHAPTER EIGHT 198

Nutritional Needs Of Children With EPI 198

Kid-Friendly Recipes............................203

CHAPTER NINE 219

Nutritional Needs Of Seniors With EPI 219

CHAPTER TEN...244

Traveling And Dining Out Tips 244

Lifestyle And Wellness Tips 250

CHAPTER ELEVEN 257

Monitoring Progress And Adjusting The Diet 257

Conclusion 264

THE END...267

Introductory

For those who suffer from exocrine pancreatic insufficiency—a disorder in which the pancreas fails to produce an adequate amount of digestive enzymes—the EPI (Exocrine Pancreatic Insufficiency) Diet is a tailored plan for nutrient absorption and digestion. The goals of this eating plan are symptom management and enhanced nutritional absorption.

Key Components of the EPI Diet:

Pancreatic Enzyme Replacement Therapy (PERT):

• Supplements containing pancreatic enzymes are taken with meals and snacks to aid digestion.

Nutrient-Dense Foods:

- Focus on foods rich in vitamins and minerals to combat nutrient deficiencies common in EPI.
- Emphasize lean proteins, fruits, vegetables, whole grains, and healthy fats.

Low-Fat Diet:

- Limit fat intake to reduce digestive strain.
- Choose lean meats, low-fat dairy, and cooking methods like baking or grilling instead of frying.

Small, Frequent Meals:

- Eating smaller, more frequent meals can help with nutrient absorption and reduce digestive discomfort.

Hydration:

- Ensure adequate fluid intake to support digestion and overall health.

Vitamin and Mineral Supplements:

- Supplements for fat-soluble vitamins (A, D, E, K) and other nutrients may be necessary.

Foods to Emphasize:

- Lean meats (chicken, turkey, fish)
- Low-fat dairy products
- Whole grains (oats, brown rice, quinoa)
- Fruits and vegetables
- Healthy fats in moderation (olive oil, avocado)

Foods to Limit:

- High-fat foods (fried foods, fatty meats)
- Processed and sugary foods

- Alcohol and caffeine (which can irritate the digestive system)

It's crucial for individuals with EPI to work with a healthcare provider, such as a gastroenterologist or a registered dietitian, to tailor the diet to their specific needs and ensure they are getting the necessary nutrients. Regular monitoring and adjustments to the diet and enzyme therapy may be needed to manage the condition effectively.

CHAPTER ONE
What Is Exocrine Pancreatic Insufficiency (EPI)

Exocrine Pancreatic Insufficiency (EPI) is a condition where the pancreas does not produce enough of the enzymes necessary for the digestion of food. These enzymes include lipase, protease, and amylase, which are essential for breaking down fats, proteins, and carbohydrates, respectively.

Causes of EPI:

- EPI can result from various underlying conditions or factors that damage the pancreas, including:

Chronic Pancreatitis:

- Long-term inflammation of the pancreas can lead to permanent damage and reduced enzyme production.

Cystic Fibrosis:

- This genetic disorder affects the exocrine glands, leading to thick mucus production that blocks the pancreatic ducts and impairs enzyme release.

Pancreatic Surgery:

- Surgical removal of part or all of the pancreas can result in EPI.

Pancreatic Cancer:

- Tumors can obstruct the pancreatic ducts or directly damage the pancreatic tissue.

Diabetes:

- Particularly type 1 diabetes, which can damage the pancreas over time.

Celiac Disease:

- This autoimmune disorder can affect the pancreas and lead to EPI.

Symptoms of EPI:

The symptoms of EPI are primarily related to malabsorption of nutrients and include:

- **Steatorrhea**: Fatty, foul-smelling stools that are difficult to flush
- **Weight Loss**: Due to poor absorption of nutrients
- **Diarrhea**: Frequent, loose, or watery stools
- **Bloating and Gas**: Caused by undigested food in the intestines

- **Abdominal Pain**: Discomfort or cramps after eating
- **Nutrient Deficiencies**: Especially fat-soluble vitamins (A, D, E, K)

Diagnosis of EPI:

Diagnosing EPI typically involves a combination of medical history, physical examination, and specific tests, such as:

- **Stool Tests**: To measure the levels of fat in the stool (fecal elastase test).
- **Blood Tests**: To check for nutrient deficiencies.
- **Imaging Studies**: Such as CT scans or MRIs to examine the pancreas.
- **Direct Pancreatic Function Tests**: Less common but can be used to measure enzyme production directly.

Treatment of EPI:

Management of EPI focuses on replacing the missing pancreatic enzymes and addressing nutritional deficiencies. Treatment typically includes:

Pancreatic Enzyme Replacement Therapy (PERT):

- Enzyme supplements are taken with meals to aid digestion.

Dietary Modifications:

- Following an EPI-friendly diet, which often includes low-fat, nutrient-dense foods.

Vitamin and Mineral Supplements:

- To address deficiencies, particularly in fat-soluble vitamins.

Managing Underlying Conditions:

- Treating the root cause of EPI, such as chronic pancreatitis or cystic fibrosis, can help manage symptoms.

Regular Monitoring:

- Ongoing evaluation by healthcare providers to adjust enzyme dosage and dietary recommendations as needed.

Macronutrients and Micronutrients:

- Macronutrients and micronutrients are essential nutrients that our bodies need to function properly, but they differ in the amounts required and their roles.

Macronutrients:

Macronutrients are nutrients that the body needs in large amounts. They provide the energy necessary for growth, metabolism, and other bodily functions. The main macronutrients are:

Carbohydrates:

- **Function**: Primary source of energy. They break down into glucose, which is used for energy by the body's cells, tissues, and organs.
- **Sources**: Fruits, vegetables, grains, legumes, and dairy products.

- **Types**: Simple carbohydrates (sugars) and complex carbohydrates (starches and fibers).

Proteins:

- **Function**: Essential for building and repairing tissues, making enzymes and hormones, and supporting immune function.

- **Sources**: Meat, poultry, fish, eggs, dairy products, legumes, nuts, seeds, and soy products.

- **Amino Acids**: Proteins are made up of amino acids, some of which are essential and must be obtained from the diet.

Fats:

- **Function**: Provide a concentrated source of energy, support cell growth, protect organs, and keep the body warm. Fats also help in the absorption of fat-soluble vitamins (A, D, E, K).

- **Sources**: Oils, butter, avocado, nuts, seeds, fatty fish, and animal products.

- **Types**: Saturated fats, unsaturated fats (monounsaturated and polyunsaturated), and trans fats (should be limited).

Micronutrients:

Micronutrients are nutrients that the body needs in smaller amounts but are crucial for proper functioning, growth, and disease prevention. They include vitamins and minerals.

Vitamins:

• **Function**: Support various bodily functions, including metabolism, immunity, and digestion. Each vitamin has specific roles in the body.

• **Types**: Water-soluble vitamins (B-complex vitamins and vitamin C) and fat-soluble vitamins (A, D, E, K).

• **Sources**: A balanced diet with a variety of foods, including fruits, vegetables, grains, dairy, and protein sources.

Minerals:

- **Function**: Essential for bone health, nerve function, muscle function, and the production of hormones and enzymes.

- **Types**: Major minerals (calcium, phosphorus, potassium, sodium, magnesium, sulfur, and chloride) and trace minerals (iron, manganese, copper, iodine, zinc, cobalt, fluoride, and selenium).

- **Sources**: Vary depending on the mineral but can include dairy products, meats, fruits, vegetables, nuts, seeds, and whole grains.

Importance of Balance:

A balanced diet that includes a variety of foods from all food groups is the best way to ensure adequate intake of both macronutrients and micronutrients. Each nutrient plays a unique role in maintaining health, and deficiencies or excesses can lead to health problems. For example:

- **Carbohydrate deficiency** can lead to low energy levels and impaired brain function.
- **Protein deficiency** can result in muscle loss and weakened immune function.
- **Fat deficiency** can affect hormone production and vitamin absorption.
- **Vitamin and mineral deficiencies** can cause a wide range of issues, from anemia (iron deficiency) to bone weakness (calcium and vitamin D deficiency).

Understanding macronutrients and micronutrients and their roles helps in planning a nutritious diet that supports overall health and well-being. It is essential to consume a variety of foods to meet the body's nutritional needs.

CHAPTER TWO
Introduction To Enzyme Replacement Therapy (ERT)

Enzyme Replacement Therapy (ERT) is a medical treatment used to replace deficient or missing enzymes in individuals with certain enzyme-related conditions. These therapies are designed to supplement the body's enzyme levels, thereby improving metabolic functions and alleviating symptoms associated with enzyme deficiencies.

Overview of Enzyme Replacement Therapy (ERT):

- **Purpose:** ERT aims to treat conditions caused by enzyme deficiencies, which can be genetic or acquired. The therapy helps in restoring normal metabolic processes and improving the quality of life for patients.

How ERT Works:

Enzyme Production:

- The deficient enzyme is produced using recombinant DNA technology or extracted from natural sources.

Administration:

- The enzyme is usually administered intravenously (IV), although some therapies may use oral or other delivery methods.

Replacement and Function:

- The administered enzyme supplements the body's natural enzyme activity, aiding in the breakdown of specific substrates and preventing the accumulation of harmful substances.

Conditions Treated with ERT:

Lysosomal Storage Disorders:

Gaucher Disease:

- Caused by a deficiency in the enzyme glucocerebrosidase.
- ERT helps break down glucocerebroside, reducing its accumulation in cells.

Fabry Disease:

- Due to a deficiency in alpha-galactosidase A.
- ERT reduces the buildup of globotriaosylceramide.

Pompe Disease:

- Caused by a deficiency in acid alpha-glucosidase.
- ERT helps break down glycogen in cells.

Exocrine Pancreatic Insufficiency (EPI):

Pancreatic Enzyme Replacement Therapy (PERT):

- Used to treat EPI, a condition where the pancreas does not produce enough digestive enzymes.
- Enzymes like lipase, protease, and amylase are supplemented to aid digestion.

Other Genetic Enzyme Deficiencies:

Mucopolysaccharidoses (MPS):

- A group of disorders caused by the deficiency of enzymes involved in glycosaminoglycan breakdown.
- ERT helps reduce the accumulation of these substances.

Benefits of ERT:

Symptom Relief:

- Reduces symptoms such as pain, organ enlargement, and other disease-specific manifestations.

Improved Quality of Life:

- Enhances overall health and well-being, enabling patients to lead more normal lives.

Preventive:

- Helps prevent or mitigate long-term complications associated with enzyme deficiencies.

Limitations and Considerations:

Accessibility and Cost:

- ERT can be expensive and may not be widely available in all regions.

Lifelong Treatment:

- Patients often require lifelong therapy to manage their conditions.

Side Effects:

- Potential for infusion-related reactions or immune responses.

Effectiveness:

- Varies depending on the condition and individual response to treatment.

Research in ERT is ongoing, with advancements aimed at improving the efficacy, delivery methods, and accessibility of treatments. Gene therapy and other innovative approaches are being explored as potential alternatives or complements to traditional ERT.

Enzyme Replacement Therapy is a crucial treatment modality for various enzyme deficiency disorders. By supplementing deficient enzymes, ERT helps restore normal metabolic functions, reduce symptoms, and improve the quality of life for affected individuals. While it presents certain challenges, ongoing research and development hold promise for enhancing the effectiveness and reach of this therapy.

Types Of Enzymes

Enzymes are biological molecules that act as catalysts to facilitate chemical reactions within the body. They are essential for numerous physiological processes, including digestion, metabolism, and cellular repair. Enzymes can be classified based on the type of reaction they catalyze. Here are the primary types of enzymes:

1. Hydrolases

- **Function**: Catalyze the hydrolysis (breaking down) of various bonds using water.

Examples:

- **Proteases**: Break down proteins into amino acids (e.g., trypsin, pepsin).

- **Lipases**: Break down fats into glycerol and fatty acids.

- **Amylases**: Break down carbohydrates into simple sugars (e.g., salivary amylase, pancreatic amylase).

2. *Oxidoreductases:*

- **Function**: Catalyze oxidation-reduction reactions, where electrons are transferred between molecules.

Examples:

- **Dehydrogenases**: Remove hydrogen atoms from substrates (e.g., lactate dehydrogenase).

- **Oxidases**: Transfer electrons to oxygen (e.g., cytochrome oxidase).

3. Transferases:

- **Function**: Transfer functional groups (e.g., methyl, phosphate) from one molecule to another.

Examples:

- **Kinases**: Transfer phosphate groups (e.g., hexokinase).

- **Transaminases**: Transfer amino groups (e.g., alanine transaminase).

4. Lyases:

- **Function**: Catalyze the addition or removal of groups to form double bonds or break down molecules without using water.

Examples:

- **Decarboxylases**: Remove carboxyl groups (e.g., pyruvate decarboxylase).

- **Aldolases**: Break down or form carbon-carbon bonds (e.g., aldolase).

5. Isomerases:

- **Function**: Catalyze the rearrangement of atoms within a molecule to form isomers.

Examples:

- **Epimerases**: Convert one isomer into another (e.g., ribose-5-phosphate isomerase).

- **Mutases**: Shift functional groups within a molecule (e.g., phosphoglucomutase).

6. Ligases:

- **Function**: Catalyze the joining of two molecules, typically using energy derived from ATP.

Examples:

- **DNA Ligase**: Joins DNA strands together during replication and repair.

- **Acetyl-CoA Synthetase**: Forms acetyl-CoA from acetate and coenzyme A.

7. Examples of Specific Enzymes and Their Functions:

- **Lactase**: Breaks down lactose into glucose and galactose, aiding in the digestion of dairy products.

- **Sucrase**: Converts sucrose into glucose and fructose.

- **Catalase**: Breaks down hydrogen peroxide into water and oxygen, protecting cells from oxidative damage.

- **Urease**: Converts urea into ammonia and carbon dioxide, playing a role in nitrogen metabolism.

Importance of Enzymes:

- **Metabolism**: Enzymes are critical for metabolic pathways, facilitating the conversion of substrates into energy and building blocks for cells.

- **Digestion**: Digestive enzymes break down food into absorbable nutrients.

- **DNA Replication and Repair**: Enzymes like DNA polymerases and ligases ensure the accuracy and integrity of genetic information.

- **Cellular Function**: Enzymes regulate cellular processes, including signal transduction, cell division, and apoptosis.

Enzyme Regulation:

- **Inhibitors**: Molecules that decrease enzyme activity. These can be competitive (competing with the substrate for the active site) or non-competitive (binding to another part of the enzyme).

- **Activators**: Molecules that increase enzyme activity.

- **Cofactors and Coenzymes**: Non-protein molecules or ions that are essential for enzyme activity. Cofactors are often metal ions, while coenzymes are organic molecules (e.g., vitamins).

Enzymes are indispensable to life's chemistry, and their study is essential for understanding and manipulating biological processes in medicine, industry, and research.

Dosage And Administration

Dosage and administration are critical aspects of any treatment plan, including enzyme replacement therapy (ERT). The correct dosage ensures the therapy's effectiveness while minimizing potential side effects. Here's an overview of how dosage and administration are approached in ERT and other contexts:

Enzyme Replacement Therapy (ERT) Dosage and Administration

1. Determining the Dosage:

• **Condition-Specific**: The dosage depends on the specific enzyme deficiency and the severity of the condition.

- **Weight-Based**: Dosages are often calculated based on the patient's weight, especially in pediatric cases.

- **Monitoring and Adjustment**: Initial dosages may be adjusted based on the patient's response, clinical symptoms, and lab results.

2. Common ERT Protocols:

Gaucher Disease:

- Typical dosages of imiglucerase (Cerezyme) range from 15 to 60 units/kg of body weight, administered every two weeks.

Fabry Disease:

- Agalsidase beta (Fabrazyme) is typically administered at a dose of 1 mg/kg every two weeks.

Pompe Disease:

- Alglucosidase alfa (Myozyme) is usually given at 20 mg/kg every two weeks.

3. Administration Methods:

Intravenous (IV) Infusion:

- Most ERTs are administered via IV infusion. The infusion time and frequency vary depending on the enzyme and the condition.

Oral Enzyme Replacement:

- Some enzymes, such as those used for exocrine pancreatic insufficiency (e.g., pancrelipase), are administered orally in capsule or tablet form with meals and snacks.

General Considerations for Dosage and Administration:

1. Individualized Treatment:

- Dosage must be tailored to the individual, taking into account factors such as age, weight, overall health, and specific medical conditions.

2. Compliance and Adherence:

- Ensuring patients follow their prescribed dosage and administration schedule is crucial for the treatment's success.

- Educating patients on the importance of adherence and providing support can help improve compliance.

3. Monitoring and Follow-Up:

• Regular monitoring of the patient's response to treatment is necessary to make any needed adjustments.

• Follow-up appointments may include physical exams, laboratory tests, and discussions about side effects or issues with the treatment regimen.

Examples of Dosage and Administration for Other Treatments:

1. Antibiotics:

• **Amoxicillin**: For adults, the typical dosage is 500 mg every 8 hours, or 875 mg every 12 hours. Pediatric dosages are weight-based.

- **Administration**: Oral tablets, capsules, or liquid suspension, taken with or without food.

2. Pain Management:

- **Ibuprofen**: For adults, the usual dosage is 200-400 mg every 4-6 hours as needed. The maximum daily dose should not exceed 3200 mg.

- **Administration**: Oral tablets, capsules, or liquid, taken with food or milk to reduce stomach irritation.

3. Chronic Conditions (e.g., Diabetes):

- **Insulin**: Dosages vary significantly based on individual blood glucose levels, diet, and activity. Insulin can be administered via injection or an insulin pump.

- **Administration**: Subcutaneous injection, typically in the abdomen, thigh, or arm.

Key Points for Safe Dosage and Administration:

- **Prescription Adherence**: Always follow the prescribed dosage and administration guidelines provided by healthcare professionals.

- **Monitoring**: Regular monitoring and consultations with healthcare providers to adjust dosages as needed.

- **Education**: Patients should be educated on the importance of following dosage instructions and aware of potential side effects.

- **Storage**: Proper storage of medications, including keeping them at the correct temperature and away from light or moisture.

- **Documentation**: Keeping a record of dosages and administration times, especially for complex regimens, can help maintain adherence and track the treatment's effectiveness.

Proper dosage and administration are critical to the success of any treatment. Tailoring the approach to individual needs, ensuring adherence, and regular monitoring are essential steps to optimize therapeutic outcomes.

CHAPTER THREE
Combining ERT With The EPI Diet

Combining Enzyme Replacement Therapy (ERT) with an Exocrine Pancreatic Insufficiency (EPI) diet is a comprehensive approach to managing EPI. This combination ensures that the body receives the necessary enzymes to aid digestion while optimizing nutrient absorption through dietary adjustments. Here's how to effectively integrate ERT with the EPI diet:

Enzyme Replacement Therapy (ERT) for EPI

Pancreatic Enzyme Replacement Therapy (PERT):

- **Purpose:** PERT provides the digestive enzymes that the pancreas fails to produce, including lipase, protease, and amylase.

- **Form:** Enzyme supplements (capsules, tablets) taken orally with meals and snacks.

- **Dosage:** Tailored based on the severity of enzyme deficiency, meal size, and fat content. Typical starting dosages are based on the patient's weight and dietary fat intake.

EPI Diet Guidelines

Nutrient-Dense Foods:

- Emphasize foods rich in vitamins and minerals to combat nutrient deficiencies.

- Include lean proteins, fruits, vegetables, whole grains, and healthy fats.

Low-Fat Diet:

- Limit fat intake to reduce digestive strain.

- Choose lean meats, low-fat dairy, and cooking methods like baking or grilling instead of frying.

Small, Frequent Meals:

- Eating smaller, more frequent meals can help with nutrient absorption and reduce digestive discomfort.

Hydration:

- Ensure adequate fluid intake to support digestion and overall health.

Vitamin and Mineral Supplements:

- Supplements for fat-soluble vitamins (A, D, E, K) and other nutrients may be necessary.

Integrating ERT with the EPI Diet

1. Timing of Enzyme Supplements:

- **With Meals and Snacks:** Take enzyme supplements at the beginning or during meals and snacks to ensure enzymes mix with food for optimal digestion.

- **Consistent Dosing:** Follow the prescribed dosage consistently, adjusting based on meal size and fat content.

2. Adjusting Diet According to Enzyme Dosage:

• **Fat Content:** Balance the fat content of meals with the enzyme dosage. Higher fat meals may require higher enzyme doses.

• **Meal Size:** Larger meals might need more enzymes, while smaller meals may require less.

3. Monitoring and Adjusting:

• **Symptom Tracking:** Monitor symptoms such as bloating, gas, and stool consistency to gauge the effectiveness of the enzyme therapy and diet.

• **Regular Consultations:** Regular check-ups with a healthcare provider to adjust enzyme dosages and dietary recommendations as needed.

4. Specific Dietary Considerations:

- **Carbohydrates:** Include complex carbohydrates like whole grains and legumes. Avoid excessive simple sugars and refined carbs.

- **Proteins:** Ensure adequate protein intake from lean sources such as poultry, fish, beans, and legumes.

- **Fats:** Focus on healthy fats in moderation, such as those from avocados, nuts, and olive oil. Avoid trans fats and limit saturated fats.

Sample Meal Plan Combining ERT and EPI Diet:

Breakfast:

- **Food:** Oatmeal with berries and a sprinkle of chia seeds.
- **ERT:** Take enzyme supplements at the beginning of the meal.

Mid-Morning Snack:

- **Food:** Greek yogurt with a small handful of almonds.
- **ERT:** Take enzyme supplements with the snack.

Lunch:

- **Food:** Grilled chicken salad with mixed greens, cherry tomatoes, cucumber, and a light vinaigrette dressing.

- **ERT:** Take enzyme supplements at the beginning of the meal.

Afternoon Snack:

- **Food:** An apple with a slice of low-fat cheese.
- **ERT:** Take enzyme supplements with the snack.

Dinner:

- **Food:** Baked salmon with quinoa and steamed broccoli.
- **ERT:** Take enzyme supplements at the beginning of the meal.

Evening Snack:

- **Food:** A small bowl of mixed berries.
- **ERT:** Take enzyme supplements with the snack if needed.

Benefits of Combining ERT with the EPI Diet:

- **Improved Digestion:** Enzymes help break down food more effectively, reducing symptoms like bloating and gas.
- **Enhanced Nutrient Absorption:** The diet ensures a good intake of essential nutrients while enzymes aid in their absorption.
- **Symptom Management:** Combined approach helps manage symptoms more effectively than diet or enzymes alone.
- **Optimized Health:** Ensures the body gets necessary nutrients while minimizing digestive discomfort.

Combining Enzyme Replacement Therapy with an EPI diet is an effective strategy to manage Exocrine Pancreatic Insufficiency. It involves taking enzyme supplements with meals and snacks, adjusting diet according to enzyme dosages, and monitoring symptoms to ensure optimal digestion and nutrient absorption. Regular consultations with healthcare providers are essential to tailor the therapy and diet to individual needs, enhancing overall health and quality of life.

Meal Planning And Preparation

Meal planning and preparation are essential for individuals managing conditions like Exocrine Pancreatic Insufficiency (EPI), where dietary choices and timing of enzyme supplements play a crucial role in digestion and overall health. Here's a guide to effective meal planning and preparation for EPI:

Meal Planning for EPI

1. Balance Macronutrients:

• **Proteins:** Lean meats (chicken, turkey), fish, tofu, legumes.

- **Carbohydrates:** Whole grains (brown rice, quinoa), fruits, vegetables.

- **Fats:** Healthy fats from avocado, nuts, seeds, and olive oil.

2. Consider Enzyme Dosage:

- Plan meals based on recommended enzyme dosages, adjusting for meal size and fat content.

3. Small, Frequent Meals:

- Opt for smaller meals throughout the day to aid digestion and nutrient absorption.

4. Nutrient-Dense Choices:

- Include foods rich in vitamins and minerals to prevent deficiencies.

5. Hydration:

- Ensure adequate fluid intake throughout the day to support digestion.

Meal Preparation Tips:

1. Preparing Enzyme Supplements:

- Take enzyme supplements at the beginning or during meals/snacks, as prescribed.

2. Cooking Methods:

- Choose cooking methods that are gentle on the digestive system, such as baking, grilling, steaming, or sautéing with minimal oil.

3. Portion Control:

- Measure portions to manage fat intake and ensure appropriate enzyme supplementation.

4. Fiber Considerations:

- Balance fiber intake to support digestive health without overwhelming enzyme activity.

5. Batch Cooking and Storage:

• Prepare meals in advance and store them in portioned containers for easy access throughout the week.

Sample Meal Ideas for EPI:

Breakfast:

• Oatmeal with sliced banana, a dollop of yogurt, and a sprinkle of chia seeds.

• Enzyme supplements taken at the beginning of the meal.

Lunch:

• Grilled chicken breast with quinoa and steamed vegetables (e.g., broccoli, carrots).

• Enzyme supplements taken before or during the meal.

Dinner:

- Baked salmon with a side of brown rice and a mixed green salad dressed with olive oil and vinegar.

- Enzyme supplements taken at the beginning of the meal.

Snacks:

- Apple slices with almond butter.

- Greek yogurt with a handful of berries.

- Enzyme supplements taken with the snack.

Benefits of Effective Meal Planning and Preparation:

- **Improved Digestion:** Proper meal planning ensures enzymes are taken with meals to aid digestion.
- **Balanced Nutrition:** Ensures a balanced intake of macronutrients and micronutrients.
- **Reduced Symptoms:** Helps manage symptoms like bloating and discomfort associated with EPI.
- **Convenience:** Preparing meals in advance saves time and ensures healthy choices are readily available.

Meal planning and preparation are integral to managing Exocrine Pancreatic Insufficiency effectively. By balancing macronutrients, considering enzyme dosage, and preparing meals with digestion in mind, individuals can optimize nutrient absorption and minimize digestive discomfort. Regular monitoring and adjustments, in consultation with healthcare providers, ensure a tailored approach that supports overall health and well-being.

CHAPTER FOUR
Breakfast Recipes

Smoothies and Shakes recipes:

Smoothies and shakes can be excellent options for individuals managing Exocrine Pancreatic Insufficiency (EPI), as they can be nutrient-dense and easily digestible. Here are some recipes for smoothies and shakes that are gentle on the digestive system and can be adjusted to fit individual dietary needs:

Basic Smoothie Guidelines for EPI:

• **Choose Low-Fat Options:** Use low-fat or non-fat dairy products (such as yogurt or milk substitutes) to reduce fat content.

• **Include Protein:** Add sources of protein like Greek yogurt, tofu, or protein powder to support muscle maintenance and repair.

- **Add Fiber Wisely:** Opt for fruits and vegetables with lower fiber content to avoid overwhelming the digestive system.

- **Enzyme Supplementation:** Take enzyme supplements with smoothies containing fats to aid digestion.

Recipes:

1. Berry Banana Smoothie:

Ingredients:

- 1 cup mixed berries (strawberries, blueberries, raspberries)
- 1 ripe banana
- 1/2 cup plain Greek yogurt (low-fat)
- 1/2 cup almond milk (or any milk substitute)
- Optional: 1 tablespoon honey or maple syrup (for sweetness)
- Ice cubes (optional)

Instructions:

- Place all ingredients in a blender.
- Blend until smooth and creamy.
- Adjust thickness with more or less liquid as desired.
- Serve immediately.

2. Tropical Green Smoothie:

Ingredients:

- 1 cup spinach or kale (packed)
- 1/2 cup frozen pineapple chunks
- 1/2 cup frozen mango chunks
- 1/2 banana
- 1/2 cup coconut water or almond milk
- Optional: 1 tablespoon chia seeds or flax seeds
- Ice cubes (optional)

Instructions:

- Combine all ingredients in a blender.

- Blend until smooth, adjusting liquid as needed.
- Taste and adjust sweetness with honey or maple syrup if desired.
- Serve immediately.

3. Peanut Butter Banana Shake:

Ingredients:

- 1 ripe banana
- 1 tablespoon natural peanut butter
- 1/2 cup plain Greek yogurt (low-fat)
- 1/2 cup almond milk (or any milk substitute)
- Optional: 1 tablespoon honey or maple syrup (for sweetness)
- Ice cubes (optional)

Instructions:

- Place all ingredients in a blender.
- Blend until smooth and creamy.

- Adjust thickness with more or less liquid as desired.
- Serve immediately.

4. Avocado Spinach Smoothie:

Ingredients:

- 1/2 ripe avocado
- 1 cup spinach (packed)
- 1/2 cup cucumber, peeled and chopped
- 1/2 cup plain Greek yogurt (low-fat)
- 1/2 cup coconut water or almond milk
- Optional: Squeeze of fresh lime juice
- Ice cubes (optional)

Instructions:

- Combine all ingredients in a blender.
- Blend until smooth, adjusting liquid as needed.
- Taste and adjust flavor with lime juice if desired.
- Serve immediately.

Tips for Adjusting Recipes:

- **Fat Content:** Adjust the amount of avocado, nut butter, or yogurt based on individual tolerance and enzyme supplementation needs.
- **Fiber Content:** Choose fruits and vegetables with lower fiber content if high fiber tends to cause discomfort.
- **Liquid Base:** Use coconut water, almond milk, or other milk substitutes for a lighter base.

Benefits of Smoothies and Shakes for EPI:

- **Nutrient Density:** Provides essential vitamins, minerals, and antioxidants in an easily digestible form.
- **Hydration:** Helps maintain hydration levels, especially with added liquids like coconut water.
- **Easy to Prepare:** Quick to make and convenient for busy schedules.
- **Variety:** Endless combinations allow for flexibility in meeting dietary needs and preferences.

Smoothies and shakes can be a versatile addition to a diet tailored for Exocrine Pancreatic Insufficiency, offering nourishment and enjoyment while supporting digestive health. Adjust ingredients based on personal preferences and consult with a healthcare provider or nutritionist for personalized guidance.

Egg-Based Dishes Recipes:

Egg-based dishes can be nutritious and versatile options for individuals managing Exocrine Pancreatic Insufficiency (EPI). Eggs are rich in protein and can be prepared in various ways that are generally well-tolerated by those with digestive concerns. Here are some simple and delicious egg-based recipes:

1. Scrambled Eggs with Spinach and Tomatoes

Ingredients:

- 2 eggs
- 1/4 cup spinach, chopped
- 1/4 cup cherry tomatoes, halved
- Salt and pepper to taste
- 1 teaspoon olive oil or butter (for cooking)

Instructions:

- Heat olive oil or butter in a non-stick skillet over medium heat.
- Whisk eggs in a bowl and season with salt and pepper.
- Pour eggs into the skillet and cook, stirring gently, until they start to set.
- Add chopped spinach and cherry tomatoes, continue cooking until eggs are fully cooked and spinach wilts.
- Serve hot.

2. Vegetable Omelette

Ingredients:

- 2 eggs
- 1/4 cup bell peppers, diced
- 1/4 cup mushrooms, sliced
- 1/4 cup spinach, chopped
- Salt and pepper to taste
- 1 teaspoon olive oil or butter (for cooking)

Instructions:

- Heat olive oil or butter in a non-stick skillet over medium heat.
- Whisk eggs in a bowl and season with salt and pepper.
- Pour eggs into the skillet and cook for a minute until the edges start to set.
- Sprinkle diced bell peppers, mushrooms, and spinach evenly over the eggs.

- Cook until the eggs are fully set and the bottom is golden brown.
- Fold the omelette in half and slide onto a plate to serve.

3. Poached Eggs with Avocado Toast

Ingredients:

- 2 eggs
- 1 ripe avocado
- 2 slices whole grain bread, toasted
- Salt and pepper to taste
- Optional: Lemon juice, red pepper flakes, or herbs for garnish

Instructions:

- Fill a saucepan with water and bring to a simmer (not boiling).
- Crack eggs into separate small bowls or ramekins.

- Gently slide each egg into the simmering water and cook for 3-4 minutes until the whites are set but the yolks are still runny.
- While eggs are cooking, mash avocado in a bowl and season with salt and pepper.
- Spread avocado evenly over toasted bread slices.
- Remove poached eggs with a slotted spoon and place on top of avocado toast.
- Season with additional salt, pepper, and optional garnishes.

4. Egg Salad Sandwich

Ingredients:

- 4 hard-boiled eggs, peeled and chopped
- 1/4 cup Greek yogurt (low-fat)
- 1 tablespoon Dijon mustard

- 1 celery stalk, finely chopped
- Salt and pepper to taste
- Whole grain bread or lettuce leaves for serving

Instructions:

- In a mixing bowl, combine chopped hard-boiled eggs, Greek yogurt, Dijon mustard, and chopped celery.
- Season with salt and pepper to taste.
- Spread egg salad mixture onto whole grain bread slices or serve in lettuce leaves for a low-carb option.
- Serve chilled or at room temperature.

Tips for Egg-Based Dishes for EPI:

- **Cooking Methods:** Opt for gentle cooking methods like scrambling, poaching, or boiling to ensure eggs are easily digestible.

- **Portion Control:** Monitor portion sizes to avoid overeating, which can strain digestion.
- **Accompaniments:** Pair with whole grain toast, vegetables, or a small portion of fruit for a balanced meal.
- **Hydration:** Drink plenty of water with meals to aid digestion and maintain hydration.

These recipes provide a variety of ways to enjoy eggs while managing Exocrine Pancreatic Insufficiency. Adjust ingredients and seasonings based on personal preferences and tolerance levels. Consulting with a healthcare provider or dietitian can help tailor meals to individual needs for optimal digestive health.

Pancakes and Waffles recipes:

Pancakes and waffles can be enjoyable and adaptable options for individuals managing Exocrine Pancreatic Insufficiency (EPI), especially when prepared with considerations for fat content and portion sizes. Here are some recipes that are gentle on the digestive system:

Pancakes

1. Basic Pancakes

Ingredients:

- 1 cup all-purpose flour (or whole wheat flour)
- 1 tablespoon sugar (optional)
- 1 teaspoon baking powder
- 1/2 teaspoon baking soda
- Pinch of salt
- 1 cup buttermilk (or milk substitute)
- 1 large egg

- 1 tablespoon melted butter or vegetable oil (plus extra for cooking)
- Optional: Vanilla extract or cinnamon for flavor

Instructions:

- In a mixing bowl, whisk together flour, sugar (if using), baking powder, baking soda, and salt.
- In another bowl, whisk together buttermilk, egg, melted butter or oil, and vanilla extract (if using).
- Pour wet ingredients into dry ingredients and stir until just combined (do not overmix).
- Heat a non-stick skillet or griddle over medium heat and lightly grease with butter or oil.
- Pour about 1/4 cup of batter onto the skillet for each pancake.

- Cook until bubbles form on the surface, then flip and cook until golden brown on both sides.
- Serve warm with toppings like fresh berries, Greek yogurt, or a drizzle of maple syrup.

2. Banana Oat Pancakes

Ingredients:

- 1 cup rolled oats
- 1 ripe banana
- 1/2 cup buttermilk (or milk substitute)
- 1 large egg
- 1 tablespoon melted butter or vegetable oil (plus extra for cooking)
- 1 teaspoon baking powder
- Pinch of salt
- Optional: Cinnamon or vanilla extract for flavor

Instructions:

- Place rolled oats in a blender or food processor and blend until finely ground (oat flour consistency).
- In a mixing bowl, mash banana and whisk together with buttermilk, egg, melted butter or oil, baking powder, salt, and optional flavorings.
- Stir in oat flour until smooth batter forms.
- Heat a non-stick skillet or griddle over medium heat and lightly grease with butter or oil.
- Pour about 1/4 cup of batter onto the skillet for each pancake.
- Cook until bubbles form on the surface, then flip and cook until golden brown on both sides.
- Serve warm with toppings of your choice.

Waffles

1. Classic Waffles

Ingredients:

- 1 1/2 cups all-purpose flour (or whole wheat flour)
- 2 tablespoons sugar (optional)
- 1 tablespoon baking powder
- 1/2 teaspoon baking soda
- Pinch of salt
- 1 1/4 cups buttermilk (or milk substitute)
- 2 large eggs
- 1/4 cup melted butter or vegetable oil
- Optional: Vanilla extract for flavor

Instructions:

- In a mixing bowl, whisk together flour, sugar (if using), baking powder, baking soda, and salt.
- In another bowl, whisk together buttermilk, eggs, melted butter or oil, and vanilla extract (if using).
- Pour wet ingredients into dry ingredients and stir until just combined (do not overmix).
- Preheat waffle iron and lightly grease with butter or oil.
- Pour appropriate amount of batter onto the preheated waffle iron (amount depends on size of waffle iron).
- Close lid and cook according to manufacturer's instructions until golden brown and crisp.
- Serve warm with toppings such as fresh fruit, yogurt, or maple syrup.

2. Whole Grain Waffles

Ingredients:

- 1 cup whole wheat flour
- 1/2 cup all-purpose flour
- 2 tablespoons sugar (optional)
- 1 tablespoon baking powder
- 1/2 teaspoon baking soda
- Pinch of salt
- 1 1/4 cups buttermilk (or milk substitute)
- 2 large eggs
- 1/4 cup melted butter or vegetable oil
- Optional: Cinnamon or nutmeg for flavor

Instructions:

- In a mixing bowl, whisk together whole wheat flour, all-purpose flour, sugar (if using), baking powder, baking soda, salt, and optional spices.

- In another bowl, whisk together buttermilk, eggs, melted butter or oil.
- Pour wet ingredients into dry ingredients and stir until just combined (do not overmix).
- Preheat waffle iron and lightly grease with butter or oil.
- Pour appropriate amount of batter onto the preheated waffle iron (amount depends on size of waffle iron).
- Close lid and cook according to manufacturer's instructions until golden brown and crisp.
- Serve warm with toppings like yogurt, fresh berries, or a drizzle of honey.

Tips for Pancakes and Waffles for EPI:

- **Fat Content:** Use melted butter or vegetable oil sparingly in recipes and consider low-fat options when possible.

- **Toppings:** Opt for fresh fruits, yogurt, or small amounts of maple syrup as toppings to minimize sugar intake.
- **Portion Control:** Monitor portion sizes to avoid overeating, which can strain digestion.
- **Accompaniments:** Serve with a side of fruit or a small portion of lean protein for a balanced meal.

These recipes offer delicious ways to enjoy pancakes and waffles while managing Exocrine Pancreatic Insufficiency. Adjust ingredients and toppings based on personal preferences and consult with a healthcare provider or dietitian for personalized guidance on dietary choices.

Cereal and Granola recipes:

Creating cereal and granola at home allows for control over ingredients, making them suitable for individuals managing Exocrine Pancreatic

Insufficiency (EPI). These recipes focus on minimizing fat content and using ingredients that are gentle on the digestive system:

Homemade Cereal

1. Oatmeal Breakfast Cereal

Ingredients:

- 2 cups rolled oats
- 1/4 cup honey or maple syrup (optional for sweetness)
- 1/4 cup chopped nuts (e.g., almonds, walnuts)
- 1/4 cup dried fruit (e.g., raisins, cranberries)
- 1 teaspoon ground cinnamon
- Pinch of salt

Instructions:

- Preheat oven to 300°F (150°C) and line a baking sheet with parchment paper.
- In a large bowl, combine rolled oats, honey or maple syrup (if using), chopped nuts, dried fruit, cinnamon, and salt. Mix well.
- Spread the mixture evenly onto the prepared baking sheet.
- Bake for 20-25 minutes, stirring halfway through, until oats are golden brown and crisp.
- Remove from oven and let cool completely before transferring to an airtight container for storage.
- Serve with milk or yogurt and fresh fruit.

2. Buckwheat and Quinoa Cereal

Ingredients:

- 1 cup buckwheat groats
- 1/2 cup quinoa, rinsed and drained
- 1/4 cup chopped nuts or seeds (e.g., sunflower seeds, pumpkin seeds)
- 1/4 cup dried fruit (e.g., chopped apricots, dried cherries)
- 2 tablespoons honey or maple syrup (optional for sweetness)
- 1 teaspoon ground cinnamon
- Pinch of salt

Instructions:

- In a dry skillet over medium heat, toast buckwheat groats and quinoa for 3-4 minutes, stirring frequently, until lightly golden and fragrant.

- Transfer toasted buckwheat and quinoa to a saucepan and add enough water to cover by about an inch.
- Bring to a boil, then reduce heat and simmer, covered, for 10-12 minutes or until grains are tender and water is absorbed.
- Remove from heat and let cool slightly.
- In a large bowl, combine cooked buckwheat and quinoa with chopped nuts or seeds, dried fruit, honey or maple syrup (if using), cinnamon, and salt. Mix well.
- Serve warm or let cool completely before storing in an airtight container.

Homemade Granola

1. Basic Honey Almond Granola

Ingredients:

- 3 cups rolled oats
- 1 cup sliced almonds
- 1/4 cup honey
- 1/4 cup melted coconut oil or vegetable oil
- 1 teaspoon vanilla extract
- 1/2 teaspoon ground cinnamon
- Pinch of salt
- 1/2 cup dried fruit (e.g., chopped dates, dried cranberries)

Instructions:

- Preheat oven to 300°F (150°C) and line a baking sheet with parchment paper.
- In a large bowl, combine rolled oats, sliced almonds, honey, melted coconut oil or vegetable oil, vanilla extract, cinnamon, and salt. Mix well until evenly coated.
- Spread the mixture evenly onto the prepared baking sheet.
- Bake for 25-30 minutes, stirring halfway through, until granola is golden brown and crisp.
- Remove from oven and let cool completely on the baking sheet.
- Stir in dried fruit and transfer to an airtight container for storage.
- Serve with milk or yogurt, or enjoy as a snack.

2. Maple Pecan Granola

Ingredients:

- 3 cups rolled oats
- 1 cup chopped pecans
- 1/4 cup maple syrup
- 1/4 cup melted butter or coconut oil
- 1 teaspoon vanilla extract
- Pinch of salt
- 1/2 cup dried fruit (e.g., chopped apricots, dried cherries)

Instructions:

- Preheat oven to 300°F (150°C) and line a baking sheet with parchment paper.
- In a large bowl, combine rolled oats, chopped pecans, maple syrup, melted butter or coconut oil, vanilla extract, and salt. Mix well until evenly coated.

- Spread the mixture evenly onto the prepared baking sheet.
- Bake for 25-30 minutes, stirring halfway through, until granola is golden brown and crisp.
- Remove from oven and let cool completely on the baking sheet.
- Stir in dried fruit and transfer to an airtight container for storage.
- Serve with milk or yogurt, or enjoy as a snack.

Tips for Cereal and Granola for EPI:

- **Fat Content:** Use minimal amounts of oil or butter and opt for lower-fat nuts and seeds.
- **Sweeteners:** Control sweetness by adjusting or omitting honey, maple syrup, or sugar based on personal preference.
- **Toppings:** Serve with milk (dairy or plant-based) or yogurt and fresh fruit for added nutrition.
- **Storage:** Store homemade cereal and granola in airtight containers at room temperature to maintain freshness.

These homemade cereal and granola recipes provide nutritious and customizable options for individuals managing Exocrine Pancreatic Insufficiency, offering control over ingredients to suit individual dietary needs and preferences. Adjust recipes as needed and consult with a healthcare provider or dietitian for personalized guidance on diet management.

CHAPTER FIVE
Lunch Recipes

Salads and Dressings recipes

Salads are excellent choices for individuals managing Exocrine Pancreatic Insufficiency (EPI) as they can be tailored to be low in fat and high in nutrients. Here are some salad and dressing recipes that are gentle on the digestive system and packed with flavor:

Salad Recipes

1. Greek Salad

Ingredients:

- 2 cups mixed salad greens (e.g., romaine lettuce, spinach)
- 1/2 cucumber, sliced
- 1/2 cup cherry tomatoes, halved
- 1/4 cup red onion, thinly sliced
- 1/4 cup Kalamata olives, pitted

- 1/4 cup feta cheese, crumbled (optional)
- Optional: Grilled chicken breast or tofu for added protein

Instructions:

- In a large salad bowl, combine mixed greens, cucumber, cherry tomatoes, red onion, and Kalamata olives.
- Top with crumbled feta cheese and grilled chicken breast or tofu if using.
- Toss gently to combine.
- Serve with a dressing of your choice.

2. Quinoa Salad

Ingredients:

- 1 cup cooked quinoa, cooled
- 1/2 cup cucumber, diced
- 1/2 cup bell peppers (any color), diced
- 1/4 cup red onion, finely chopped

- 1/4 cup fresh parsley, chopped
- 1/4 cup crumbled feta cheese (optional)
- Optional: Grilled shrimp or chickpeas for added protein

Instructions:

- In a large bowl, combine cooked quinoa, cucumber, bell peppers, red onion, and fresh parsley.
- Add crumbled feta cheese and grilled shrimp or chickpeas if using.
- Toss gently to mix all ingredients evenly.
- Serve chilled or at room temperature.

Dressing Recipes

1. Lemon Herb Vinaigrette

Ingredients:

- 1/4 cup extra virgin olive oil

- 2 tablespoons fresh lemon juice
- 1 teaspoon Dijon mustard
- 1 garlic clove, minced
- 1 tablespoon fresh herbs (e.g., basil, parsley), finely chopped
- Salt and pepper to taste

Instructions:

- In a small bowl, whisk together olive oil, lemon juice, Dijon mustard, minced garlic, and fresh herbs.
- Season with salt and pepper to taste.
- Use immediately or store in a sealed container in the refrigerator for up to one week.

2. Greek Yogurt Ranch Dressing

Ingredients:

- 1/2 cup plain Greek yogurt (low-fat)
- 2 tablespoons fresh lemon juice

- 1 tablespoon chopped fresh dill
- 1 tablespoon chopped fresh parsley
- 1 garlic clove, minced
- Salt and pepper to taste

Instructions:

- In a bowl, whisk together Greek yogurt, lemon juice, chopped dill, chopped parsley, and minced garlic.
- Season with salt and pepper to taste.
- Adjust consistency with a little water if needed.
- Serve immediately or refrigerate in a sealed container for up to one week.

Tips for Salads and Dressings for EPI:

- **Leafy Greens:** Use tender greens like spinach or mixed baby greens to ease digestion.
- **Protein:** Add lean protein sources like grilled chicken breast, tofu, or beans for satiety and muscle maintenance.
- **Fats:** Opt for healthy fats in moderation such as olive oil or avocado to aid nutrient absorption.
- **Portion Control:** Monitor serving sizes to avoid overeating and strain on digestion.

These salad and dressing recipes provide nutritious and flavorful options for individuals managing Exocrine Pancreatic Insufficiency, promoting digestive health while enjoying satisfying meals.

Adjust ingredients and flavors based on personal preferences and consult with a healthcare provider or dietitian for personalized dietary recommendations.

Soups and Stews recipes:

Soups and stews can be comforting and nourishing options for individuals managing Exocrine Pancreatic Insufficiency (EPI), especially when prepared with ingredients that are easy to digest and low in fat. Here are some gentle recipes that focus on flavor and nutrient density:

Soup Recipes

1. Chicken and Rice Soup

Ingredients:

- 1 tablespoon olive oil
- 1 small onion, diced
- 2 carrots, diced
- 2 celery stalks, diced
- 1 garlic clove, minced
- 4 cups low-sodium chicken broth or vegetable broth
- 1 cup cooked chicken breast, shredded

- 1/2 cup cooked rice
- Salt and pepper to taste
- Fresh parsley or dill for garnish

Instructions:

- In a large pot, heat olive oil over medium heat.
- Add diced onion, carrots, and celery. Cook until vegetables are softened, about 5-7 minutes.
- Add minced garlic and cook for another minute until fragrant.
- Pour in chicken broth and bring to a simmer.
- Add shredded chicken breast and cooked rice to the pot.
- Season with salt and pepper to taste.
- Simmer for 10-15 minutes to allow flavors to meld.
- Serve hot, garnished with fresh parsley or dill.

2. Lentil and Vegetable Soup

Ingredients:

- 1 tablespoon olive oil
- 1 small onion, diced
- 2 carrots, diced
- 2 celery stalks, diced
- 1 cup dried lentils, rinsed and drained
- 4 cups low-sodium vegetable broth or chicken broth
- 1 teaspoon ground cumin
- 1 teaspoon paprika
- Salt and pepper to taste
- Fresh parsley for garnish

Instructions:

- In a large pot, heat olive oil over medium heat.
- Add diced onion, carrots, and celery. Cook until vegetables are softened, about 5-7 minutes.

- Add rinsed lentils, broth, ground cumin, and paprika to the pot.
- Bring to a boil, then reduce heat to low and simmer, covered, for 20-25 minutes or until lentils are tender.
- Season with salt and pepper to taste.
- Serve hot, garnished with fresh parsley.

Stew Recipes

1. Beef and Vegetable Stew

Ingredients:

- 1 tablespoon olive oil
- 1 pound beef stew meat, cut into bite-sized pieces
- 1 onion, diced
- 2 carrots, diced
- 2 celery stalks, diced
- 2 garlic cloves, minced

- 4 cups low-sodium beef broth or vegetable broth
- 1 cup diced tomatoes (canned or fresh)
- 1 teaspoon dried thyme
- Salt and pepper to taste
- Fresh parsley for garnish

Instructions:

- In a large pot or Dutch oven, heat olive oil over medium-high heat.
- Add beef stew meat and brown on all sides, about 5-7 minutes.
- Add diced onion, carrots, celery, and minced garlic. Cook until vegetables are softened, about 5 minutes.
- Pour in beef broth, diced tomatoes, and dried thyme. Bring to a boil.
- Reduce heat to low, cover, and simmer for 1 to 1.5 hours or until beef is tender.
- Season with salt and pepper to taste.

- Serve hot, garnished with fresh parsley.

2. Potato and Leek Soup

Ingredients:

- 2 tablespoons unsalted butter or olive oil
- 2 leeks, white and light green parts only, thinly sliced
- 2 large potatoes, peeled and diced
- 4 cups low-sodium vegetable broth or chicken broth
- 1/2 cup whole milk or cream (optional)
- Salt and pepper to taste
- Fresh chives for garnish

Instructions:

- In a large pot, melt butter over medium heat (or heat olive oil).

- Add sliced leeks and cook until softened, about 5-7 minutes.
- Add diced potatoes and broth to the pot. Bring to a boil.
- Reduce heat to low, cover, and simmer for 15-20 minutes or until potatoes are tender.
- Use an immersion blender to puree the soup until smooth (or transfer to a blender in batches).
- Stir in whole milk or cream if using, and season with salt and pepper to taste.
- Serve hot, garnished with fresh chives.

Tips for Soups and Stews for EPI:

- **Fat Content:** Use lean cuts of meat and minimal amounts of oil or butter.
- **Vegetables:** Choose well-cooked and easily digestible vegetables like carrots, celery, and potatoes.

- **Broth:** Opt for low-sodium broth to control salt intake.
- **Portion Control:** Enjoy in moderate portions to avoid overeating and strain on digestion.

These soup and stew recipes offer hearty and nourishing options for individuals managing Exocrine Pancreatic Insufficiency, providing comfort and essential nutrients. Adjust ingredients and flavors based on personal preferences and consult with a healthcare provider or dietitian for personalized dietary recommendations.

Sandwiches and Wraps recipes:

Sandwiches and wraps can be versatile and satisfying options for individuals managing Exocrine Pancreatic Insufficiency (EPI), especially when using ingredients that are easy to digest and low in fat. Here are some gentle and flavorful recipes:

Sandwich Recipes

1. Turkey and Avocado Sandwich

Ingredients:

- 2 slices whole grain bread (or bread of choice)
- 2-3 slices roasted turkey breast
- 1/4 avocado, sliced
- Leafy greens (e.g., spinach, lettuce)
- Optional: Sliced tomato, cucumber

Instructions:

- Toast the bread slices lightly if desired.
- Layer roasted turkey breast, sliced avocado, leafy greens, and any additional vegetables on one slice of bread.
- Top with the second slice of bread.
- Cut in half diagonally and serve.

2. Egg Salad Sandwich

Ingredients:

- 2 slices whole grain bread (or bread of choice)
- 2 hard-boiled eggs, chopped
- 2 tablespoons plain Greek yogurt (low-fat)
- 1 teaspoon Dijon mustard
- Salt and pepper to taste
- Leafy greens (e.g., spinach, lettuce)
- Optional: Sliced tomato, cucumber

Instructions:

- In a bowl, mix chopped hard-boiled eggs with Greek yogurt, Dijon mustard, salt, and pepper.
- Toast the bread slices lightly if desired.
- Spread egg salad mixture evenly on one slice of bread.

- Top with leafy greens, sliced tomato, cucumber, and the second slice of bread.
- Cut in half diagonally and serve.

Wrap Recipes:

1. Chicken and Hummus Wrap

Ingredients:

- 1 large whole wheat tortilla wrap
- 1/2 cup cooked chicken breast, shredded or sliced
- 2 tablespoons hummus (flavor of choice)
- 1/4 cup shredded carrots
- 1/4 cup baby spinach leaves
- Optional: Sliced cucumber, bell peppers

Instructions:

- Lay the tortilla wrap flat on a plate or cutting board.
- Spread hummus evenly over the tortilla.
- Layer cooked chicken breast, shredded carrots, baby spinach leaves, and any additional vegetables down the center of the wrap.
- Roll the tortilla tightly, folding in the sides as you go.
- Slice in half diagonally and serve.

2. Veggie and Avocado Wrap:

Ingredients:

- 1 large whole wheat tortilla wrap
- 1/2 avocado, mashed
- 1/4 cup hummus (flavor of choice)
- 1/4 cup shredded carrots
- 1/4 cup cucumber, thinly sliced
- 1/4 cup baby spinach leaves

- Optional: Sliced bell peppers, sprouts

Instructions:

- Lay the tortilla wrap flat on a plate or cutting board.
- Spread mashed avocado and hummus evenly over the tortilla.
- Layer shredded carrots, cucumber slices, baby spinach leaves, and any additional vegetables down the center of the wrap.
- Roll the tortilla tightly, folding in the sides as you go.
- Slice in half diagonally and serve.

Tips for Sandwiches and Wraps for EPI:

- **Bread and Wraps:** Choose whole grain bread or wraps for added fiber and easier digestion.
- **Protein:** Opt for lean protein sources like turkey, chicken breast, or eggs.

- **Vegetables:** Include fresh, crunchy vegetables that are easy to chew and digest.
- **Condiments:** Use minimal amounts of condiments and spreads to control fat and calorie intake.
- **Portion Control:** Enjoy in moderate portions to avoid overeating and strain on digestion.

These sandwich and wrap recipes offer nutritious and satisfying meal options for individuals managing Exocrine Pancreatic Insufficiency, providing variety and essential nutrients without compromising on taste.

Adjust ingredients and flavors based on personal preferences and consult with a healthcare provider or dietitian for personalized dietary recommendations.

Grain Bowls recipes:

Grain bowls are nutritious and versatile options for individuals managing Exocrine Pancreatic Insufficiency (EPI), providing a balanced meal with whole grains, lean proteins, and vegetables. Here are some grain bowl recipes that are gentle on digestion and packed with flavor:

Quinoa and Vegetable Bowl:

Ingredients:

- 1 cup cooked quinoa
- 1/2 cup cooked chickpeas (canned, rinsed and drained)
- 1/2 cup steamed or roasted vegetables (e.g., broccoli, bell peppers, zucchini)
- 1/4 cup diced cucumber
- 1/4 cup cherry tomatoes, halved
- 1/4 avocado, sliced
- Fresh herbs for garnish (e.g., parsley, cilantro)

- Optional: Grilled chicken breast or tofu cubes

Instructions:

- Cook quinoa according to package instructions and let cool slightly.
- Arrange cooked quinoa in a bowl as the base.
- Top with cooked chickpeas, steamed or roasted vegetables, diced cucumber, cherry tomatoes, and sliced avocado.
- Add grilled chicken breast or tofu cubes if using.
- Garnish with fresh herbs.
- Serve warm or at room temperature.

Brown Rice and Salmon Bowl:

Ingredients:

- 1 cup cooked brown rice

- 4 oz grilled or baked salmon fillet, flaked
- 1/2 cup steamed or sautéed spinach
- 1/4 cup shredded carrots
- 1/4 cup edamame (shelled)
- 1/4 cup sliced cucumber
- Lemon wedges for garnish
- Optional: Soy sauce or tamari for drizzling

Instructions:

- Cook brown rice according to package instructions and let cool slightly.
- Arrange cooked brown rice in a bowl as the base.
- Top with flaked salmon, steamed or sautéed spinach, shredded carrots, edamame, and sliced cucumber.
- Drizzle with soy sauce or tamari if desired.
- Garnish with lemon wedges.

- Serve warm or at room temperature.

Mediterranean Quinoa Bowl

Ingredients:

- 1 cup cooked quinoa
- 1/2 cup diced cooked chicken breast or grilled tofu cubes
- 1/4 cup cherry tomatoes, halved
- 1/4 cup cucumber, diced
- 1/4 cup Kalamata olives, pitted and sliced
- 2 tablespoons crumbled feta cheese
- Fresh parsley for garnish
- Optional: Lemon vinaigrette or Greek yogurt dressing

Instructions:

- Cook quinoa according to package instructions and let cool slightly.
- Arrange cooked quinoa in a bowl as the base.

- Top with diced chicken breast or grilled tofu cubes, cherry tomatoes, cucumber, Kalamata olives, and crumbled feta cheese.
- Drizzle with lemon vinaigrette or Greek yogurt dressing if using.
- Garnish with fresh parsley.
- Serve warm or at room temperature.

Tips for Grain Bowls for EPI:

- **Grains:** Choose whole grains like quinoa, brown rice, or barley for added fiber and easier digestion.
- **Proteins:** Opt for lean proteins such as grilled chicken breast, tofu, or fish to minimize fat content.
- **Vegetables:** Include a variety of steamed, roasted, or raw vegetables for texture and nutrients.

- **Seasonings:** Use herbs, lemon juice, or light dressings for flavor instead of heavy sauces.
- **Portion Control:** Enjoy in moderate portions to prevent overeating and support digestive comfort.

These grain bowl recipes offer nutritious and balanced meal options for individuals managing Exocrine Pancreatic Insufficiency, promoting digestion-friendly ingredients while providing essential nutrients and flavors. Adjust ingredients and seasonings based on personal preferences and consult with a healthcare provider or dietitian for personalized dietary recommendations.

CHAPTER SIX
Dinner Recipes

Poultry and Meat Dishes recipes:

Here are some gentle and flavorful poultry and meat dish recipes suitable for individuals managing Exocrine Pancreatic Insufficiency (EPI). These recipes focus on lean cuts of meat and minimal fat content:

Grilled Chicken Breast with Lemon and Herbs

Ingredients:

- 2 boneless, skinless chicken breasts
- 2 tablespoons fresh lemon juice
- 2 garlic cloves, minced
- 1 tablespoon olive oil
- 1 teaspoon dried herbs (such as thyme, rosemary, or oregano)
- Salt and pepper to taste

Instructions:

- In a bowl, whisk together lemon juice, minced garlic, olive oil, dried herbs, salt, and pepper.
- Place chicken breasts in a shallow dish or resealable plastic bag. Pour the marinade over the chicken, turning to coat evenly.
- Marinate in the refrigerator for at least 30 minutes (or up to 4 hours for more flavor).
- Preheat grill to medium-high heat. Grill chicken breasts for 6-8 minutes per side, or until internal temperature reaches 165°F (75°C).
- Remove from grill and let rest for a few minutes before slicing.
- Serve hot, garnished with fresh herbs if desired.

Turkey and Vegetable Stir-Fry

Ingredients:

- 1 lb turkey breast or tenderloin, thinly sliced
- 2 tablespoons soy sauce (low-sodium)
- 1 tablespoon rice vinegar
- 1 tablespoon honey
- 1 tablespoon sesame oil
- 2 garlic cloves, minced
- 1 teaspoon fresh ginger, minced
- 1 cup broccoli florets
- 1 bell pepper, sliced
- 1 carrot, sliced
- 1/2 cup snow peas
- Cooked brown rice or quinoa for serving

Instructions:

- In a small bowl, whisk together soy sauce, rice vinegar, honey, sesame oil, minced garlic, and minced ginger.
- Heat a large skillet or wok over medium-high heat. Add turkey slices

and stir-fry until browned and cooked through, about 5-7 minutes. Remove turkey from skillet and set aside.
- In the same skillet, add broccoli florets, bell pepper slices, carrot slices, and snow peas. Stir-fry for 3-4 minutes, or until vegetables are tender-crisp.
- Return cooked turkey to the skillet. Pour the sauce over the turkey and vegetables, stirring to coat evenly.
- Cook for another 1-2 minutes until heated through and sauce has thickened slightly.
- Serve immediately over cooked brown rice or quinoa.

Beef and Vegetable Stir-Fry

Ingredients:

- 1 lb beef sirloin or flank steak, thinly sliced

- 2 tablespoons low-sodium soy sauce
- 1 tablespoon hoisin sauce
- 1 tablespoon rice vinegar
- 1 tablespoon cornstarch
- 1 tablespoon vegetable oil
- 2 garlic cloves, minced
- 1 teaspoon fresh ginger, minced
- 1 cup broccoli florets
- 1 bell pepper, sliced
- 1 carrot, sliced
- Cooked rice noodles or brown rice for serving

Instructions:

- In a bowl, whisk together soy sauce, hoisin sauce, rice vinegar, and cornstarch until smooth.
- Heat vegetable oil in a large skillet or wok over medium-high heat. Add minced garlic and minced ginger,

- stirring for about 30 seconds until fragrant.
- Add beef slices to the skillet and stir-fry until browned, about 3-4 minutes.
- Add broccoli florets, bell pepper slices, and carrot slices to the skillet. Stir-fry for another 3-4 minutes, or until vegetables are tender-crisp.
- Pour the sauce over the beef and vegetables, stirring to coat evenly. Cook for another 1-2 minutes until sauce has thickened slightly.
- Serve immediately over cooked rice noodles or brown rice.

Tips for Poultry and Meat Dishes for EPI:

• **Lean Cuts:** Choose lean cuts of poultry and meat to reduce fat content.

• **Marination:** Marinate poultry and meat with citrus juices, herbs, and spices to enhance flavor without adding fat.

- **Cooking Methods:** Opt for grilling, baking, or stir-frying with minimal oil to reduce fat intake.

- **Portion Control:** Enjoy in moderate portions to support digestion and prevent discomfort.

These poultry and meat dish recipes provide delicious and digestion-friendly options for individuals managing Exocrine Pancreatic Insufficiency, offering balanced nutrition and satisfying flavors.

Adjust ingredients and seasonings based on personal preferences and consult with a healthcare provider or dietitian for personalized dietary recommendations.

Seafood and Fish recipes:

Here are some gentle and flavorful seafood and fish recipes suitable for individuals managing Exocrine Pancreatic Insufficiency

(EPI). These recipes focus on lean proteins and minimal fat content:

Grilled Salmon with Lemon and Dill:

Ingredients:

- 2 salmon fillets (about 6 oz each), skin-on or skinless
- 2 tablespoons fresh lemon juice
- 2 tablespoons olive oil
- 1 tablespoon fresh dill, chopped (or 1 teaspoon dried dill)
- Salt and pepper to taste

Instructions:

- In a small bowl, whisk together lemon juice, olive oil, chopped dill, salt, and pepper.
- Place salmon fillets in a shallow dish or resealable plastic bag. Pour the marinade over the salmon, turning to coat evenly.

- Marinate in the refrigerator for at least 30 minutes (or up to 2 hours for more flavor).
- Preheat grill to medium-high heat. Grill salmon fillets, skin-side down if using skin-on, for 4-5 minutes. Carefully flip and grill for another 3-4 minutes, or until salmon flakes easily with a fork and internal temperature reaches 145°F (63°C).
- Remove from grill and let rest for a few minutes before serving.
- Serve hot, garnished with additional fresh dill and lemon wedges if desired.

Shrimp Stir-Fry with Vegetables:

Ingredients:

- 1 lb large shrimp, peeled and deveined
- 2 tablespoons low-sodium soy sauce
- 1 tablespoon rice vinegar
- 1 tablespoon honey

- 1 tablespoon sesame oil
- 1 garlic clove, minced
- 1 teaspoon fresh ginger, minced
- 1 cup broccoli florets
- 1 bell pepper, sliced
- 1 carrot, sliced
- 1/2 cup snow peas
- Cooked brown rice or quinoa for serving

Instructions:

- In a bowl, whisk together soy sauce, rice vinegar, honey, sesame oil, minced garlic, and minced ginger.
- Heat a large skillet or wok over medium-high heat. Add shrimp and stir-fry until pink and cooked through, about 3-4 minutes. Remove shrimp from skillet and set aside.
- In the same skillet, add broccoli florets, bell pepper slices, carrot slices,

- and snow peas. Stir-fry for 3-4 minutes, or until vegetables are tender-crisp.
- Return cooked shrimp to the skillet. Pour the sauce over the shrimp and vegetables, stirring to coat evenly.
- Cook for another 1-2 minutes until heated through and sauce has thickened slightly.
- Serve immediately over cooked brown rice or quinoa.

Baked Cod with Herbs and Lemon:

Ingredients:

- 2 cod fillets (about 6 oz each)
- 2 tablespoons fresh lemon juice
- 2 tablespoons olive oil
- 1 tablespoon fresh parsley, chopped
- 1 teaspoon dried dill
- Salt and pepper to taste

Instructions:

- Preheat oven to 400°F (200°C). Lightly grease a baking dish with olive oil or line with parchment paper.
- In a small bowl, whisk together lemon juice, olive oil, chopped parsley, dried dill, salt, and pepper.
- Place cod fillets in the prepared baking dish. Pour the herb and lemon mixture over the cod, spreading evenly to coat.
- Bake for 12-15 minutes, or until cod flakes easily with a fork and reaches an internal temperature of 145°F (63°C).
- Remove from oven and let rest for a few minutes before serving.
- Serve hot, garnished with additional fresh herbs and lemon wedges if desired.

Tips for Seafood and Fish Recipes for EPI:

- **Lean Choices:** Choose lean seafood and fish options such as salmon, shrimp, cod, or tilapia to reduce fat content.
- **Marination:** Marinate seafood with citrus juices, herbs, and spices to enhance flavor without adding fat.
- **Cooking Methods:** Opt for grilling, baking, or stir-frying with minimal oil to reduce fat intake.
- **Portion Control:** Enjoy in moderate portions to support digestion and prevent discomfort.

These seafood and fish recipes provide delicious and digestion-friendly options for individuals managing Exocrine Pancreatic Insufficiency, offering balanced nutrition and satisfying flavors. Adjust ingredients and seasonings based on personal preferences and consult with a healthcare provider or dietitian for personalized dietary recommendations.

Vegetarian and Vegan Options recipes:

Here are some delicious and digestion-friendly vegetarian and vegan recipes suitable for individuals managing Exocrine Pancreatic Insufficiency (EPI). These recipes focus on plant-based ingredients that are easy to digest and packed with nutrients:

Quinoa and Black Bean Stuffed Bell Peppers (Vegan)

Ingredients:

- 4 large bell peppers, any color
- 1 cup quinoa, rinsed
- 1 can (15 oz) black beans, rinsed and drained
- 1 cup corn kernels (fresh, frozen, or canned)
- 1 small onion, diced
- 2 garlic cloves, minced
- 1 teaspoon ground cumin

- 1 teaspoon chili powder
- Salt and pepper to taste
- Fresh cilantro for garnish
- Optional: Salsa or avocado slices for serving

Instructions:

- Preheat oven to 375°F (190°C). Lightly grease a baking dish with olive oil or cooking spray.
- Cut the tops off the bell peppers and remove seeds and membranes. Place the peppers upright in the prepared baking dish.
- Cook quinoa according to package instructions and set aside.
- In a large skillet, heat olive oil over medium heat. Add diced onion and cook until softened, about 5 minutes.

- Add minced garlic, ground cumin, and chili powder. Cook for another minute until fragrant.
- Stir in black beans, corn kernels, and cooked quinoa. Season with salt and pepper to taste. Cook for 2-3 minutes until heated through.
- Spoon the quinoa and black bean mixture evenly into the bell peppers.
- Cover the baking dish with foil and bake for 25-30 minutes, or until bell peppers are tender.
- Remove from oven and let cool slightly before serving.
- Garnish with fresh cilantro and serve with salsa or avocado slices if desired.

Chickpea and Vegetable Curry (Vegan):

Ingredients:

- 1 tablespoon coconut oil or olive oil
- 1 onion, diced

- 2 garlic cloves, minced
- 1 tablespoon fresh ginger, minced
- 1 tablespoon curry powder
- 1 teaspoon ground cumin
- 1/2 teaspoon turmeric powder
- 1 can (15 oz) chickpeas, rinsed and drained
- 1 can (14 oz) diced tomatoes
- 1 can (14 oz) coconut milk (full-fat or light)
- 2 cups chopped vegetables (e.g., bell peppers, carrots, spinach)
- Salt and pepper to taste
- Fresh cilantro for garnish
- Cooked brown rice or quinoa for serving

Instructions:

- In a large pot or deep skillet, heat coconut oil over medium heat.

- Add diced onion and cook until softened, about 5 minutes.
- Add minced garlic and minced ginger. Cook for another minute until fragrant.
- Stir in curry powder, ground cumin, and turmeric powder. Cook for 1-2 minutes until spices are toasted.
- Add chickpeas, diced tomatoes (with juices), and coconut milk to the pot. Stir to combine.
- Bring the mixture to a simmer. Cover and cook for 15-20 minutes, stirring occasionally, until vegetables are tender.
- Season with salt and pepper to taste.
- Serve hot over cooked brown rice or quinoa.
- Garnish with fresh cilantro before serving.

Lentil and Vegetable Soup (Vegetarian):

Ingredients:

- 1 tablespoon olive oil
- 1 onion, diced
- 2 carrots, diced
- 2 celery stalks, diced
- 1 cup dried green or brown lentils, rinsed and drained
- 4 cups low-sodium vegetable broth or water
- 1 can (14 oz) diced tomatoes
- 1 teaspoon dried thyme
- Salt and pepper to taste
- Fresh parsley for garnish

Instructions:

- In a large pot, heat olive oil over medium heat.
- Add diced onion, carrots, and celery. Cook until vegetables are softened, about 5-7 minutes.

- Add rinsed lentils, vegetable broth or water, diced tomatoes (with juices), and dried thyme to the pot.
- Bring to a boil, then reduce heat to low and simmer, covered, for 30-40 minutes or until lentils are tender.
- Season with salt and pepper to taste.
- Serve hot, garnished with fresh parsley.

Tips for Vegetarian and Vegan Options for EPI:

- **Protein Sources:** Include plant-based proteins such as beans, lentils, chickpeas, and tofu.
- **Vegetables:** Use a variety of colorful vegetables that are easy to digest, such as bell peppers, spinach, carrots, and broccoli.
- **Herbs and Spices:** Use herbs and spices to add flavor without adding fat or salt.
- **Whole Grains:** Serve with whole grains like brown rice, quinoa, or whole grain bread for added fiber and nutrients.

These vegetarian and vegan recipes provide nutritious and flavorful options for individuals managing Exocrine Pancreatic Insufficiency, supporting digestive comfort while ensuring balanced nutrition. Adjust ingredients and seasonings based on personal preferences and consult with a healthcare provider or dietitian for personalized dietary recommendations.

Side Dishes recipes:

Here are some gentle and flavorful side dish recipes suitable for individuals managing Exocrine Pancreatic Insufficiency (EPI). These recipes focus on using ingredients that are easy to digest and packed with nutrients:

Roasted Garlic Mashed Potatoes

Ingredients:

- 1 lb Yukon Gold potatoes, peeled and cut into chunks
- 2-3 garlic cloves, peeled
- 2 tablespoons olive oil
- Salt and pepper to taste
- 1/4 cup low-fat milk or vegetable broth (optional)

Instructions:

- Preheat oven to 400°F (200°C).
- Place potato chunks and peeled garlic cloves on a baking sheet. Drizzle with olive oil and season with salt and pepper.
- Toss to coat evenly and spread out in a single layer.
- Roast in the oven for 25-30 minutes, or until potatoes are tender and lightly golden, flipping halfway through.
- Transfer roasted potatoes and garlic to a bowl. Mash with a potato masher or fork until desired consistency.
- If needed, add low-fat milk or vegetable broth gradually to achieve desired creaminess.
- Season with additional salt and pepper if necessary.
- Serve hot as a side dish.

Quinoa Salad with Lemon Vinaigrette

Ingredients:

- 1 cup quinoa, rinsed
- 1 1/2 cups water or vegetable broth
- 1 cucumber, diced
- 1 bell pepper, diced
- 1/4 cup red onion, finely chopped
- 1/4 cup fresh parsley, chopped
- 1/4 cup feta cheese, crumbled (optional)
- Salt and pepper to taste

For Lemon Vinaigrette:

- 1/4 cup olive oil
- 2 tablespoons fresh lemon juice
- 1 teaspoon Dijon mustard
- 1 garlic clove, minced
- Salt and pepper to taste

Instructions:

- In a medium saucepan, bring water or vegetable broth to a boil. Add quinoa, reduce heat to low, cover, and simmer for 15-20 minutes, or until liquid is absorbed and quinoa is tender. Remove from heat and let cool slightly.
- In a large bowl, combine cooked quinoa, diced cucumber, diced bell pepper, chopped red onion, and chopped parsley.
- In a small bowl or jar, whisk together olive oil, lemon juice, Dijon mustard, minced garlic, salt, and pepper to make the vinaigrette.
- Pour the vinaigrette over the quinoa salad and toss to coat evenly.
- If using, sprinkle crumbled feta cheese over the salad.
- Season with additional salt and pepper if needed.

- Serve chilled or at room temperature.

Steamed Green Beans with Almonds:

Ingredients:

- 1 lb green beans, trimmed
- 2 tablespoons sliced almonds
- 1 tablespoon olive oil
- Salt and pepper to taste
- Lemon wedges for serving

Instructions:

- Steam green beans until tender-crisp, about 5-7 minutes.
- While green beans are steaming, heat olive oil in a small skillet over medium heat.
- Add sliced almonds and toast, stirring frequently, until lightly golden and fragrant, about 2-3 minutes. Be careful not to burn.
- Remove almonds from heat and set aside.

- Once green beans are cooked, transfer them to a serving dish.
- Drizzle with olive oil, season with salt and pepper to taste.
- Sprinkle toasted almonds over the green beans.
- Serve hot with lemon wedges on the side.

Tips for Side Dishes for EPI:

- **Fiber Content:** Choose side dishes with moderate fiber content to support digestive comfort.
- **Cooking Methods:** Opt for steaming, roasting, or light sautéing with minimal added fats.
- **Flavor Enhancers:** Use herbs, spices, and citrus juices to add flavor without adding excessive fats or sugars.
- **Portion Control:** Enjoy side dishes in moderate portions to complement

main meals without overwhelming digestion.

These side dish recipes provide nutritious and digestion-friendly options for individuals managing Exocrine Pancreatic Insufficiency, offering balanced nutrition and satisfying flavors. Adjust ingredients and seasonings based on personal preferences and consult with a healthcare provider or dietitian for personalized dietary recommendations.

CHAPTER SEVEN
Snack And Dessert Recipes

Healthy Snacks recipes:

Here are some healthy and digestion-friendly snack recipes suitable for individuals managing Exocrine Pancreatic Insufficiency (EPI). These snacks are nutrient-dense and easy to digest:

Hummus with Crudites:

Ingredients:

- 1 can (15 oz) chickpeas, rinsed and drained
- 2 tablespoons tahini (sesame seed paste)
- 2 tablespoons fresh lemon juice
- 1 garlic clove, minced
- 2 tablespoons olive oil
- Salt and pepper to taste
- Assorted raw vegetables for dipping (e.g., baby carrots, cucumber slices, bell pepper strips)

Instructions:

- In a food processor, combine chickpeas, tahini, fresh lemon juice, minced garlic, olive oil, salt, and pepper.
- Process until smooth and creamy, adding a tablespoon of water if needed to achieve desired consistency.

- Transfer hummus to a serving bowl.
- Arrange assorted raw vegetables on a platter for dipping.
- Serve hummus with crudites for a nutritious snack.

Greek Yogurt with Berries and Honey:

Ingredients:

- 1 cup plain Greek yogurt
- 1/2 cup mixed berries (e.g., strawberries, blueberries, raspberries)
- 1 tablespoon honey or maple syrup
- Optional: Chopped nuts or seeds for topping

Instructions:

- Spoon Greek yogurt into a bowl.
- Top with mixed berries.
- Drizzle with honey or maple syrup.
- Sprinkle with chopped nuts or seeds if desired.

- Serve immediately for a refreshing and protein-packed snack.

Rice Cake with Almond Butter and Banana Slices

Ingredients:

- 1 rice cake (choose whole grain for added fiber)
- 1 tablespoon almond butter (or any nut butter of choice)
- 1/2 banana, thinly sliced

Instructions:

- Spread almond butter evenly on the rice cake.
- Arrange banana slices on top.
- Enjoy as a quick and satisfying snack.

Baked Sweet Potato Chips

Ingredients:

- 1 large sweet potato, thinly sliced into rounds
- 1 tablespoon olive oil
- Salt and pepper to taste

Instructions:

- Preheat oven to 375°F (190°C). Line a baking sheet with parchment paper.
- In a bowl, toss sweet potato slices with olive oil, salt, and pepper until evenly coated.
- Arrange sweet potato slices in a single layer on the prepared baking sheet.
- Bake for 15-20 minutes, flipping halfway through, until chips are crispy and lightly browned.
- Remove from oven and let cool slightly before serving.
- Enjoy baked sweet potato chips as a crunchy and nutritious snack.

Tips for Healthy Snacks for EPI:

- **Fiber Content:** Choose snacks with moderate fiber content to support digestive comfort.
- **Protein:** Incorporate snacks with protein to help stabilize blood sugar levels and provide sustained energy.
- **Hydration:** Stay hydrated by pairing snacks with water or herbal teas.
- **Portion Control:** Enjoy snacks in moderate portions to prevent discomfort and support digestion.

These healthy snack recipes provide nutritious and digestion-friendly options for individuals managing Exocrine Pancreatic Insufficiency, offering balanced nutrition and satisfying flavors. Adjust ingredients and portion sizes based on personal preferences and consult with a healthcare provider or dietitian for personalized dietary recommendations.

Baked Goods recipes:

Here are some baked goods recipes that are gentle on digestion and suitable for individuals managing Exocrine Pancreatic Insufficiency (EPI). These recipes focus on using ingredients that are low in fat and easy to digest:

Banana Oat Muffins:

Ingredients:

- 1 cup oats (quick or old-fashioned)
- 1 cup whole wheat flour or oat flour
- 1 teaspoon baking powder
- 1/2 teaspoon baking soda
- 1/4 teaspoon salt
- 2 ripe bananas, mashed
- 1/2 cup plain Greek yogurt
- 1/4 cup honey or maple syrup
- 1/4 cup milk (dairy or non-dairy)
- 1 egg
- 1 teaspoon vanilla extract

- Optional add-ins: 1/2 cup chopped nuts, dried fruit, or chocolate chips

Instructions:

- Preheat oven to 350°F (175°C). Line a muffin tin with paper liners or lightly grease with oil.
- In a large bowl, combine oats, whole wheat flour (or oat flour), baking powder, baking soda, and salt.
- In another bowl, whisk together mashed bananas, Greek yogurt, honey (or maple syrup), milk, egg, and vanilla extract until smooth.
- Pour wet ingredients into dry ingredients and stir until just combined. Do not overmix.
- If using, fold in chopped nuts, dried fruit, or chocolate chips.
- Divide batter evenly among muffin cups, filling each about 3/4 full.

- Bake for 18-20 minutes, or until a toothpick inserted into the center comes out clean.
- Remove from oven and let cool in the pan for 5 minutes before transferring to a wire rack to cool completely.
- Enjoy banana oat muffins as a wholesome snack or breakfast option.

Low-Fat Blueberry Scones:

Ingredients:

- 2 cups whole wheat flour
- 1/4 cup sugar
- 2 teaspoons baking powder
- 1/2 teaspoon baking soda
- 1/4 teaspoon salt
- 1/4 cup cold unsalted butter, cut into small pieces
- 1 cup fresh or frozen blueberries
- 1/2 cup plain Greek yogurt
- 1/4 cup milk (dairy or non-dairy)

- 1 egg
- 1 teaspoon vanilla extract

Instructions:

- Preheat oven to 400°F (200°C). Line a baking sheet with parchment paper.
- In a large bowl, whisk together whole wheat flour, sugar, baking powder, baking soda, and salt.
- Cut in cold butter pieces using a pastry cutter or fork until mixture resembles coarse crumbs.
- Gently fold in blueberries.
- In a separate bowl, whisk together Greek yogurt, milk, egg, and vanilla extract until smooth.
- Pour wet ingredients into dry ingredients and stir until just combined. Do not overmix.

- Transfer dough onto a lightly floured surface and gently knead a few times until dough comes together.
- Pat dough into a circle about 1-inch thick. Cut into 8 wedges.
- Place scones on the prepared baking sheet. Bake for 15-18 minutes, or until scones are lightly golden and cooked through.
- Remove from oven and let cool on a wire rack for a few minutes before serving.
- Enjoy low-fat blueberry scones warm or at room temperature.

Applesauce Oatmeal Cookies:

Ingredients:

- 1 cup oats (quick or old-fashioned)
- 1 cup whole wheat flour or oat flour
- 1/2 teaspoon baking soda
- 1/2 teaspoon ground cinnamon

- 1/4 teaspoon salt
- 1/4 cup unsweetened applesauce
- 1/4 cup honey or maple syrup
- 1/4 cup unsalted butter, melted and cooled
- 1 egg
- 1 teaspoon vanilla extract
- 1/2 cup raisins or dried cranberries (optional)

Instructions:

- Preheat oven to 350°F (175°C). Line a baking sheet with parchment paper.
- In a large bowl, combine oats, whole wheat flour (or oat flour), baking soda, ground cinnamon, and salt.
- In another bowl, whisk together applesauce, honey (or maple syrup), melted butter, egg, and vanilla extract until smooth.

- Pour wet ingredients into dry ingredients and stir until just combined. Do not overmix.
- If using, fold in raisins or dried cranberries.
- Drop tablespoon-sized mounds of dough onto the prepared baking sheet, spacing them about 2 inches apart.
- Flatten each mound slightly with the back of a spoon or fork.
- Bake for 10-12 minutes, or until cookies are lightly golden around the edges.
- Remove from oven and let cool on the baking sheet for 5 minutes before transferring to a wire rack to cool completely.
- Enjoy applesauce oatmeal cookies as a healthier treat.

Tips for Baked Goods for EPI:

- **Low-Fat Ingredients:** Use minimal amounts of unsaturated fats like olive oil or unsalted butter.
- **Fruit and Fiber:** Incorporate fruits, whole grains, and oats for added fiber and nutrients.
- **Sweeteners:** Opt for natural sweeteners such as honey, maple syrup, or applesauce instead of refined sugars.
- **Portion Control:** Enjoy in moderation to support digestion and prevent discomfort.

These baked goods recipes provide nutritious and digestion-friendly options for individuals managing Exocrine Pancreatic Insufficiency, offering balanced nutrition and comforting flavors. Adjust ingredients and portion sizes based on personal preferences and consult with a healthcare provider or dietitian for personalized dietary recommendations.

Fruits and Smoothies recipes:

Here are some gentle and digestion-friendly fruit recipes and smoothie ideas suitable for individuals managing Exocrine Pancreatic Insufficiency (EPI). These recipes focus on using fruits that are easy to digest and packed with nutrients:

Fresh Fruit Salad

Ingredients:

- 1 cup fresh strawberries, hulled and sliced
- 1 cup fresh blueberries
- 1 cup fresh pineapple, diced
- 1 cup seedless grapes, halved
- 1 banana, sliced
- Optional: Fresh mint leaves for garnish

Instructions:

- Combine all prepared fruits in a large bowl.
- Gently toss to mix.
- Serve immediately or chill in the refrigerator until ready to serve.
- Garnish with fresh mint leaves if desired.

Digestive Smoothie

Ingredients:

- 1 cup plain Greek yogurt
- 1/2 cup fresh or frozen berries (e.g., strawberries, blueberries, raspberries)
- 1/2 banana
- 1 tablespoon ground flaxseed or chia seeds
- 1/2 cup spinach leaves (optional)
- 1/2 cup water or unsweetened almond milk

Instructions:

- Place all ingredients in a blender.
- Blend until smooth and creamy, adding more water or almond milk if needed to reach desired consistency.
- Pour into a glass and serve immediately.

Tropical Papaya Smoothie:

Ingredients:

- 1 cup fresh papaya, diced
- 1/2 cup fresh pineapple, diced
- 1/2 banana
- 1/2 cup coconut water or plain water
- Juice of 1/2 lime
- Optional: 1 tablespoon honey or maple syrup (if additional sweetness is desired)

Instructions:

- Combine papaya, pineapple, banana, coconut water (or plain water), lime

juice, and optional sweetener in a blender.
- Blend until smooth and creamy.
- Pour into a glass and serve immediately.

Banana Oat Smoothie:

Ingredients:

- 1 ripe banana
- 1/2 cup rolled oats
- 1/2 cup plain Greek yogurt
- 1 tablespoon honey or maple syrup
- 1/2 teaspoon vanilla extract
- 1/2 cup water or unsweetened almond milk
- Ice cubes (optional)

Instructions:

- Place banana, rolled oats, Greek yogurt, honey (or maple syrup),

vanilla extract, and water (or almond milk) in a blender.
- Add ice cubes if desired for a colder smoothie.
- Blend until smooth and creamy.
- Pour into a glass and serve immediately.

Tips for Fruits and Smoothies for EPI:

- **Choose Easy-to-Digest Fruits:** Opt for fruits such as berries, bananas, papaya, and pineapple that are generally gentle on digestion.
- **Include Fiber:** Incorporate sources of soluble fiber like oats, flaxseed, or chia seeds to support digestive health.
- **Hydration:** Smoothies can help with hydration, especially when made with coconut water or plain water.
- **Avoid Excess Sugars:** Limit added sugars and opt for natural sweeteners

like honey or maple syrup in moderation.

These fruit recipes and smoothie ideas provide nutritious and digestion-friendly options for individuals managing Exocrine Pancreatic Insufficiency, offering refreshing flavors and essential nutrients. Adjust ingredients based on personal preferences and consult with a healthcare provider or dietitian for personalized dietary recommendations.

Desserts recipes:

Here are some gentle and digestion-friendly dessert recipes suitable for individuals managing Exocrine Pancreatic Insufficiency (EPI). These recipes focus on using ingredients that are low in fat and easy to digest:

Fruit and Yogurt Parfait:

Ingredients:

- 1 cup plain Greek yogurt
- 1 tablespoon honey or maple syrup (optional, adjust to taste)
- 1/2 cup fresh berries (e.g., strawberries, blueberries, raspberries)
- 1/4 cup granola (choose low-fat and low-sugar varieties)
- Optional: Sliced bananas or other fruits of choice

Instructions:

- In a bowl, mix plain Greek yogurt with honey or maple syrup (if using), until well combined.
- In a glass or bowl, layer Greek yogurt mixture, fresh berries, and granola.
- Repeat layers until ingredients are used up, ending with a layer of yogurt on top.
- Garnish with additional berries or sliced fruits if desired.
- Serve immediately or refrigerate until ready to enjoy.

Chia Seed Pudding

Ingredients:

- 1/4 cup chia seeds
- 1 cup unsweetened almond milk or coconut milk

- 1 tablespoon honey or maple syrup (optional, adjust to taste)
- 1/2 teaspoon vanilla extract
- Fresh berries or fruit slices for topping

Instructions:

- In a bowl or jar, combine chia seeds, almond milk (or coconut milk), honey or maple syrup (if using), and vanilla extract. Stir well.
- Cover and refrigerate for at least 2 hours, or overnight, until mixture thickens and becomes pudding-like consistency.
- Stir again before serving.
- Serve chilled, topped with fresh berries or fruit slices.

Baked Apples with Cinnamon:

Ingredients:

- 2 apples (such as Fuji or Gala), cored

- 1 tablespoon honey or maple syrup
- 1/2 teaspoon ground cinnamon
- Optional: Chopped nuts (e.g., walnuts or almonds)

Instructions:

- Preheat oven to 375°F (190°C).
- In a small bowl, mix honey or maple syrup with ground cinnamon until well combined.
- Place cored apples on a baking sheet lined with parchment paper.
- Spoon cinnamon mixture into the center of each apple.
- Optional: Sprinkle chopped nuts over the top of the apples.
- Bake for 20-25 minutes, or until apples are tender and lightly golden.
- Remove from oven and let cool slightly before serving.
- Serve warm as a comforting dessert.

Mango Sorbet:

Ingredients:

- 2 cups frozen mango chunks
- 1/4 cup coconut water or plain water
- 1 tablespoon honey or maple syrup (optional, adjust to taste)
- Juice of 1/2 lime

Instructions:

- Place frozen mango chunks, coconut water (or plain water), honey or maple syrup (if using), and lime juice in a blender or food processor.
- Blend until smooth and creamy, scraping down the sides as needed.
- If mixture is too thick, add more coconut water or water a little at a time until desired consistency is reached.

- Serve immediately as soft serve, or transfer to a container and freeze for 1-2 hours for a firmer sorbet.
- Scoop mango sorbet into bowls and enjoy.

Tips for Desserts for EPI:

- **Low-Fat Options:** Choose desserts with minimal added fats and oils.
- **Natural Sweeteners:** Use honey, maple syrup, or fruits to add sweetness instead of refined sugars.
- **Fruit Focus:** Incorporate fruits which are generally easier to digest.
- **Portion Control:** Enjoy desserts in moderation to support digestion and prevent discomfort.

These dessert recipes provide nutritious and digestion-friendly options for individuals managing Exocrine Pancreatic Insufficiency, offering satisfying flavors and essential nutrients. Adjust ingredients based on personal preferences and consult with a healthcare provider or dietitian for personalized dietary recommendations.

CHAPTER EIGHT
Nutritional Needs Of Children With EPI

Children with Exocrine Pancreatic Insufficiency (EPI) have specific nutritional needs to ensure they receive adequate nutrients and support optimal growth and development. Here are some key considerations:

Macronutrients:

• **Protein:** Essential for growth and repair. Choose lean sources such as poultry, fish, beans, and dairy (if tolerated).

• **Carbohydrates:** Provide energy. Opt for whole grains like oats, brown rice, and whole wheat bread to aid digestion with their fiber content.

- **Fats:** Important for energy and fat-soluble vitamin absorption. Use healthy fats like olive oil, avocados, and nuts.

Micronutrients:

- **Vitamins:** Especially vitamins A, D, E, and K which are fat-soluble and may require supplementation or careful monitoring in EPI.

- **Minerals:** Ensure adequate intake of calcium, iron, zinc, and magnesium, which are crucial for bone health, immune function, and overall growth.

Dietary Guidelines:

- **Enzyme Replacement Therapy (ERT):** Administer enzymes with all meals and snacks to aid in the digestion and absorption of nutrients.

- **Balanced Meals:** Encourage regular, balanced meals and snacks to maintain stable blood sugar levels and support digestion.

- **Hydration:** Ensure adequate fluid intake to support digestion and prevent dehydration, especially if diarrhea is a concern.

- **Monitor Growth:** Regularly track growth parameters (height, weight, BMI) to ensure adequate nutrition and adjust dietary intake as needed.

Work closely with a healthcare provider or dietitian to tailor a nutrition plan specific to the child's needs, considering their age, growth stage, and any other health conditions.

Sample Meal Ideas For Kids:

- **Breakfast:** Whole grain toast with nut butter, banana slices, and a glass of fortified milk.
- **Lunch:** Grilled chicken or tofu with quinoa and steamed vegetables.
- **Snack:** Greek yogurt with berries and a sprinkle of granola.
- **Dinner:** Baked fish with sweet potato wedges and a side of mixed greens.

Dietary Adjustments:

- **Low-Fat Approach:** Minimize high-fat foods to reduce the burden on pancreatic function.
- **Small, Frequent Meals:** Offer smaller portions more frequently throughout the day to aid digestion and optimize nutrient absorption.

By focusing on nutrient-dense foods, supporting enzyme replacement therapy, and monitoring growth and dietary intake, caregivers can help children with EPI thrive nutritionally and developmentally. Always consult healthcare professionals for personalized advice and guidance.

Kid-Friendly Recipes

Here are some kid-friendly recipes that are gentle on digestion and suitable for children managing Exocrine Pancreatic Insufficiency (EPI). These recipes are nutritious, easy to prepare, and incorporate ingredients that are generally well-tolerated:

Turkey and Vegetable Meatballs:

Ingredients:

- 1 lb ground turkey (or chicken)
- 1/2 cup grated zucchini
- 1/2 cup grated carrot
- 1/4 cup finely chopped spinach
- 1/4 cup breadcrumbs (choose whole wheat for added fiber)
- 1 egg
- 1/2 teaspoon garlic powder
- 1/2 teaspoon onion powder
- Salt and pepper to taste

- Olive oil for cooking

Instructions:

- Preheat oven to 375°F (190°C). Line a baking sheet with parchment paper.
- In a large bowl, combine ground turkey, grated zucchini, grated carrot, chopped spinach, breadcrumbs, egg, garlic powder, onion powder, salt, and pepper. Mix until well combined.
- Shape mixture into small meatballs and place them on the prepared baking sheet.
- Lightly brush or spray meatballs with olive oil.
- Bake for 20-25 minutes, or until meatballs are cooked through and lightly browned.
- Serve warm with a side of whole grain pasta or steamed vegetables.

Mini Veggie Quesadillas:

Ingredients:

- Whole wheat tortillas (small size)
- 1/2 cup shredded cheddar cheese (or cheese of choice)
- 1/4 cup finely chopped bell peppers (red, green, or yellow)
- 1/4 cup corn kernels (fresh or canned, drained)
- 1/4 cup black beans (rinsed and drained)
- Olive oil for cooking

Instructions:

- Heat a non-stick skillet over medium heat.
- Place a tortilla in the skillet and sprinkle with shredded cheese.
- Top half of the tortilla with chopped bell peppers, corn kernels, and black beans.

- Fold the tortilla in half over the filling, pressing down gently with a spatula.
- Cook for 2-3 minutes on each side, or until tortilla is golden brown and cheese is melted.
- Remove from skillet and let cool slightly before slicing into wedges.
- Serve warm with salsa or guacamole for dipping.

Banana Oat Pancakes:

Ingredients:

- 1 cup oats (quick or old-fashioned)
- 1 ripe banana
- 1/2 cup plain Greek yogurt
- 1/4 cup milk (dairy or non-dairy)
- 1 egg
- 1 teaspoon vanilla extract
- 1/2 teaspoon ground cinnamon
- 1/2 teaspoon baking powder
- Olive oil or butter for cooking

Instructions:

- In a blender or food processor, combine oats, ripe banana, Greek yogurt, milk, egg, vanilla extract, ground cinnamon, and baking powder. Blend until smooth.
- Heat a non-stick skillet or griddle over medium heat. Lightly grease with olive oil or butter.
- Pour pancake batter onto the skillet to form pancakes of desired size.
- Cook for 2-3 minutes, or until bubbles form on the surface of the pancakes. Flip and cook for another 1-2 minutes, or until golden brown and cooked through.
- Repeat with remaining batter.
- Serve warm with a drizzle of honey or maple syrup and fresh fruit slices.

Fruit and Yogurt Popsicles:

Ingredients:

- 1 cup plain Greek yogurt
- 1 tablespoon honey or maple syrup
- 1 cup mixed berries (e.g., strawberries, blueberries, raspberries)
- Optional: Sliced bananas or other fruits of choice

Instructions:

- In a bowl, mix plain Greek yogurt with honey or maple syrup until well combined.
- Gently fold in mixed berries and optional sliced bananas.
- Spoon mixture into popsicle molds.
- Insert popsicle sticks and freeze for at least 4 hours, or until firm.
- To remove popsicles from molds, briefly run under warm water.
- Serve frozen as a refreshing treat.

Tips for Kid-Friendly Recipes for EPI:

- **Texture:** Consider the texture of foods—choose softer textures and finely chopped ingredients to aid digestion.
- **Small Portions:** Offer smaller portions to prevent overwhelming digestion and allow for better nutrient absorption.
- **Hydration:** Encourage regular water intake throughout the day, especially if fiber-rich foods are included.

These kid-friendly recipes provide nutritious options that are gentle on digestion for children managing Exocrine Pancreatic Insufficiency. Adjust ingredients based on individual preferences and consult with healthcare providers or dietitians for personalized dietary recommendations.

Tips for Parents and Caregivers:

Managing Exocrine Pancreatic Insufficiency (EPI) in children requires attention to their dietary needs, digestive health, and overall well-being. Here are some tips for parents and caregivers to support children with EPI:

1. Educate Yourself

- **Understand EPI:** Learn about the condition, its symptoms, and how it affects digestion and nutrient absorption.

- **Treatment Options:** Familiarize yourself with Enzyme Replacement Therapy (ERT), its administration, and its role in managing EPI.

2. Work with Healthcare Providers

- **Consult Specialists:** Regularly visit pediatricians, gastroenterologists, and dietitians who have experience with EPI.

- **Customized Care:** Work with healthcare providers to develop a personalized treatment plan, including enzyme dosing, dietary adjustments, and monitoring growth.

3. Optimize Nutrition

- **Balanced Diet:** Ensure children receive a balanced diet rich in nutrients, including proteins, carbohydrates, fats, vitamins, and minerals.

- **Digestion-Friendly Foods:** Choose easily digestible foods such as lean proteins, whole grains, fruits, and vegetables.

4. Meal Planning

- **Regular Meals:** Establish regular meal times and encourage consistent eating habits to support digestion and nutrient absorption.

- **Portion Control:** Offer smaller, more frequent meals and snacks to prevent overwhelming the digestive system.

5. Enzyme Replacement Therapy (ERT)

- **Consistent Administration:** Administer pancreatic enzyme supplements with all meals and snacks as prescribed.

- **Adjust as Needed:** Monitor effectiveness and adjust enzyme dosage based on food intake, symptoms, and growth.

6. Hydration:

- **Encourage Water Intake:** Ensure children drink an adequate amount of water throughout the day to support digestion and prevent dehydration.

7. Monitor Symptoms:

- **Observe Digestive Symptoms:** Keep track of symptoms such as abdominal pain, bloating, diarrhea, or weight loss. Report any changes to healthcare providers promptly.

- **Growth Monitoring:** Regularly monitor growth parameters (height, weight, BMI) to assess nutritional status and adjust dietary intake as needed.

8. Supportive Environment:

- **Open Communication:** Create an open and supportive environment where children feel comfortable discussing their symptoms and dietary preferences.

- **Educate Family Members:** Educate family members, caregivers, and school personnel about EPI and the child's dietary needs.

9. Emotional Support:

• **Encourage Independence:** Support children in managing their condition independently as they grow older, including enzyme administration and food choices.

• **Emotional Well-Being:** Address any emotional challenges related to living with a chronic condition and provide encouragement and reassurance.

10. Stay Informed and Engaged:

• **Stay Updated:** Keep up-to-date with new research, treatment options, and support resources for EPI.

• **Support Networks:** Connect with other parents, caregivers, and support groups for shared experiences and advice.

By actively managing diet, administering enzyme replacement therapy as prescribed, monitoring symptoms and growth, and providing emotional support, parents and caregivers can effectively support children with Exocrine Pancreatic Insufficiency.

Collaboration with healthcare providers is essential for developing and adjusting a comprehensive care plan tailored to the child's individual needs and ensuring optimal health and well-being.

CHAPTER NINE
Nutritional Needs Of Seniors With EPI

Seniors with Exocrine Pancreatic Insufficiency (EPI) require careful attention to their nutritional needs to maintain health, manage symptoms, and support overall well-being. Here are some key considerations for addressing the nutritional needs of seniors with EPI:

Macronutrients:

Protein:

- **Importance:** Essential for muscle maintenance and repair.

- **Sources:** Lean meats (e.g., poultry, fish), low-fat dairy (if tolerated), eggs, legumes, and plant-based proteins like tofu.

Carbohydrates:

- **Importance:** Provide energy and fiber for digestive health.

- **Sources:** Whole grains (e.g., oats, whole wheat), fruits, vegetables, and legumes.

Fats:

- **Importance:** Necessary for energy and absorption of fat-soluble vitamins.

- **Sources:** Healthy fats such as olive oil, avocados, nuts, and seeds. Limit saturated and trans fats.

Micronutrients:

Vitamins:

- **Fat-Soluble Vitamins:** Vitamin A, D, E, and K may require supplementation or careful monitoring due to impaired fat digestion.

- **Water-Soluble Vitamins:** B vitamins (especially B12) and vitamin C are important for energy production, nerve function, and immune health.

Minerals:

- **Calcium:** Essential for bone health. Sources include dairy products (if tolerated), fortified non-dairy milks, and leafy green vegetables.

- **Magnesium, Zinc, and Iron:** Support various bodily functions and may require attention to ensure adequate intake.

Dietary Guidelines:

Enzyme Replacement Therapy (ERT):

- **Importance:** Administer enzymes with all meals and snacks to aid in the digestion and absorption of nutrients.

- **Dosage:** Adjust enzyme dosage based on meal size and fat content to optimize digestion.

Balanced Meals:

- **Nutrient Density:** Encourage nutrient-dense foods to meet nutritional needs without overloading the digestive system.

- **Fiber:** Include soluble fiber from fruits, vegetables, and whole grains to support digestive health.

Hydration:

- **Importance:** Ensure seniors drink adequate fluids throughout the day to prevent dehydration and support digestion.

Regular Monitoring:

- **Symptoms:** Monitor for symptoms such as abdominal pain, bloating, diarrhea, or unintentional weight loss, and adjust diet and enzyme therapy as needed.

- **Nutritional Status:** Regularly assess nutritional status and consult healthcare providers for guidance on dietary adjustments.

Sample Meal Ideas:

- **Breakfast:** Greek yogurt with granola and berries, scrambled eggs with spinach, whole grain toast.

- **Lunch:** Grilled chicken or tofu salad with mixed greens, quinoa, and vegetables.

- **Dinner:** Baked fish with steamed vegetables and quinoa or brown rice.

Dietary Adjustments

- **Low-Fat Diet:** Minimize high-fat foods to reduce the burden on pancreatic function and optimize digestion.

- **Small, Frequent Meals:** Offer smaller portions more frequently throughout the day to aid digestion and nutrient absorption.

Tips for Seniors with EPI:

- **Individualized Care:** Tailor dietary recommendations to meet individual needs, considering health conditions, medications, and personal preferences.

- **Meal Planning:** Plan meals and snacks in advance to ensure balanced nutrition and adequate enzyme administration.

- **Consultation:** Work closely with healthcare providers, including dietitians, to develop and adjust a nutrition plan specific to the senior's needs and monitor for any changes in health or digestion.

By focusing on nutrient-dense foods, supporting enzyme replacement therapy, and monitoring symptoms and nutritional status, caregivers and healthcare providers can help seniors with Exocrine Pancreatic Insufficiency maintain optimal health and quality of life. Regular communication with healthcare providers is crucial for adapting dietary strategies as needed to meet evolving health needs.

Easy-to-Prepare Recipes for seniors:

Here are some easy-to-prepare and digestion-friendly recipes suitable for seniors, particularly those managing Exocrine Pancreatic Insufficiency (EPI). These recipes are gentle on digestion, nutrient-dense, and designed to be simple to make:

1. Vegetable and Chicken Stir-Fry

Ingredients:

- 1 tablespoon olive oil
- 1 boneless, skinless chicken breast, thinly sliced
- 1 cup broccoli florets
- 1 bell pepper, thinly sliced
- 1 carrot, thinly sliced
- 1/2 onion, thinly sliced
- 2 cloves garlic, minced
- 2 tablespoons low-sodium soy sauce

- Cooked brown rice or quinoa, for serving

Instructions:

- Heat olive oil in a large skillet or wok over medium-high heat.
- Add sliced chicken breast and cook until browned and cooked through, about 5-7 minutes.
- Add broccoli, bell pepper, carrot, onion, and minced garlic to the skillet. Stir-fry for another 5 minutes or until vegetables are tender-crisp.
- Stir in low-sodium soy sauce and cook for 1-2 minutes more.
- Serve stir-fry over cooked brown rice or quinoa.

2. *Creamy Tomato Basil Soup*

Ingredients:

- 1 tablespoon olive oil

- 1 onion, diced
- 2 cloves garlic, minced
- 1 can (28 oz) diced tomatoes
- 1 cup low-sodium vegetable or chicken broth
- 1/2 cup plain Greek yogurt or coconut milk (for dairy-free option)
- 1/4 cup fresh basil leaves, chopped
- Salt and pepper to taste

Instructions:

- Heat olive oil in a large pot over medium heat.
- Add diced onion and minced garlic. Cook until softened, about 5 minutes.
- Stir in diced tomatoes (with juices) and broth. Bring to a simmer and cook for 10-15 minutes.
- Use an immersion blender to puree the soup until smooth. Alternatively, transfer soup in batches to a blender

and blend until smooth. Be cautious with hot liquids.
- Stir in Greek yogurt or coconut milk and chopped basil. Season with salt and pepper to taste.
- Serve warm, optionally garnished with additional basil leaves.

3. Baked Lemon Herb Salmon

Ingredients:

- 2 salmon fillets (6 oz each)
- 1 tablespoon olive oil
- 1 lemon, thinly sliced
- 2 cloves garlic, minced
- 1 teaspoon dried thyme
- Salt and pepper to taste

Instructions:

- Preheat oven to 400°F (200°C). Line a baking sheet with parchment paper.

- Place salmon fillets on the prepared baking sheet.
- Drizzle olive oil over salmon fillets. Rub minced garlic and dried thyme evenly onto each fillet.
- Arrange lemon slices over the salmon.
- Bake for 12-15 minutes, or until salmon flakes easily with a fork and internal temperature reaches 145°F (63°C).
- Serve warm with steamed vegetables or a side salad.

4. Greek Yogurt Parfait with Berries and Almonds

Ingredients:

- 1 cup plain Greek yogurt
- 1 tablespoon honey or maple syrup (optional)
- 1/2 cup mixed berries (e.g., strawberries, blueberries, raspberries)

- 2 tablespoons sliced almonds

Instructions:

- In a bowl or glass, layer plain Greek yogurt and drizzle with honey or maple syrup if desired.
- Add mixed berries on top of yogurt.
- Sprinkle sliced almonds over the berries.
- Serve immediately as a nutritious snack or light dessert.

5. Avocado and Tomato Salad

Ingredients:

- 1 ripe avocado, diced
- 1 cup cherry tomatoes, halved
- 1/4 cup red onion, thinly sliced
- 2 tablespoons fresh cilantro or parsley, chopped
- Juice of 1/2 lemon
- 1 tablespoon olive oil

- Salt and pepper to taste

Instructions:

- In a salad bowl, combine diced avocado, cherry tomatoes, red onion, and chopped cilantro or parsley.
- Drizzle lemon juice and olive oil over the salad.
- Season with salt and pepper to taste.
- Toss gently to combine.
- Serve immediately as a refreshing side dish.

Tips for Seniors:

• **Preparation:** Choose recipes with minimal preparation and cooking time to reduce stress and effort.

• **Texture:** Consider softer textures and finely chopped ingredients to aid digestion.

- **Nutrient Density:** Opt for nutrient-dense foods to meet nutritional needs without overwhelming the digestive system.

These recipes provide nutritious and easy-to-prepare options for seniors managing Exocrine Pancreatic Insufficiency, promoting both health and enjoyment in mealtime. Adjust ingredients based on individual preferences and consult with healthcare providers or dietitians for personalized dietary recommendations.

Tips for Caregivers:

Caring for someone with Exocrine Pancreatic Insufficiency (EPI) involves understanding their specific needs related to diet, medication, and overall health. Here are some practical tips for caregivers to support individuals with EPI:

1. Education and Awareness:

- **Learn About EPI:** Understand the causes, symptoms, and treatment options for EPI. This knowledge helps in providing informed care and support.

- **Stay Updated:** Keep abreast of new research, medications, and dietary guidelines related to EPI to ensure the best care possible.

2. Collaborate with Healthcare Providers:

- **Regular Check-ups:** Ensure the person under your care attends regular medical appointments with gastroenterologists, dietitians, and other specialists as needed.

- **Follow Treatment Plans:** Adhere to prescribed medications, such as pancreatic enzyme replacement therapy (ERT), and monitor their effectiveness. Report any changes or concerns to healthcare providers promptly.

3. Nutritional Support:

- **Balanced Diet:** Work with a dietitian to create a balanced meal plan that meets the individual's nutritional needs while considering the challenges of EPI, such as fat malabsorption.

- **Enzyme Replacement Therapy (ERT):** Administer pancreatic enzymes with all meals and snacks as directed. Ensure proper dosage based on the amount of food and its fat content.

4. Meal Preparation and Planning:

• **Digestion-Friendly Foods:** Choose foods that are low in fat, easily digestible, and rich in nutrients. Consider softer textures and finely chopped ingredients to aid digestion.

• **Meal Timing:** Encourage regular meal times and smaller, more frequent meals throughout the day to support digestion and nutrient absorption.

5. Monitor Symptoms and Adjust Care:

• **Symptom Management:** Monitor for symptoms such as abdominal pain, bloating, diarrhea, or unintended weight loss. Keep a record of symptoms to share with healthcare providers.

• **Medication Adherence:** Ensure the person takes prescribed medications consistently and at the correct times. Help with organizing medications if needed.

6. Emotional and Social Support:

• **Encourage Independence:** Support the individual in managing their condition independently whenever possible, such as administering their own enzymes and making food choices.

• **Provide Emotional Support:** Living with a chronic condition can be challenging. Offer empathy, encouragement, and reassurance to help maintain emotional well-being.

7. Hydration and Lifestyle Factors:

• **Hydration:** Encourage adequate fluid intake throughout the day to support digestion and prevent dehydration, especially during episodes of diarrhea.

• **Physical Activity:** Promote gentle physical activity as appropriate, which can aid digestion and overall health. Consult with healthcare providers for exercise recommendations.

8. Practical Considerations:

• **Meal Preparation Tips:** Use meal prep techniques to make cooking easier, such as preparing ingredients in advance and using kitchen tools that simplify cooking tasks.

• **Safety and Comfort:** Ensure the environment is safe and comfortable for meal preparation and eating, considering any mobility or sensory challenges the individual may have.

9. Stay Organized and Communicate:

• **Documentation:** Keep a record of medications, dietary preferences, and medical appointments. This helps in coordinating care and providing accurate information to healthcare providers.

• **Open Communication:** Foster open communication with the person you are caring for, their healthcare team, and other involved caregivers or family members. Collaboration ensures comprehensive care and support.

10. Self-Care for Caregivers:

- **Take Breaks:** Caregiving can be demanding. Take regular breaks to rest, recharge, and maintain your own well-being.

- **Seek Support:** Don't hesitate to seek support from support groups, counseling services, or respite care services to manage caregiver stress and burnout effectively.

By following these tips, caregivers can provide effective support and improve the quality of life for individuals living with Exocrine Pancreatic Insufficiency. Each person's needs may vary, so adapting care strategies and seeking professional guidance as needed is crucial for personalized care.

CHAPTER TEN
Traveling And Dining Out Tips

Traveling and dining out can present unique challenges for individuals managing Exocrine Pancreatic Insufficiency (EPI) due to the need for careful meal planning and management of enzyme replacement therapy (ERT). Here are some tips to help navigate these situations effectively:

Traveling Tips:

Plan Ahead:

- Research restaurants and grocery stores at your destination that offer suitable options for your dietary needs.

- Pack enough enzyme supplements and medications for the duration of your trip, plus extra in case of delays.

Communicate Needs:

- Notify airlines or transportation services in advance if you require special meals or have dietary restrictions.

- Inform hotel staff about your dietary needs to ensure they can accommodate you during your stay.

Pack Smart:

- Carry snacks that are low in fat and easy to digest, such as crackers, rice cakes, or dried fruits.

- Pack a small cooler bag with perishable snacks like yogurt cups or sliced fruits if traveling by car.

Stay Hydrated:

• Drink plenty of water during travel to stay hydrated, especially if flying or in dry climates.

Stay Organized:

• Keep medications and enzyme supplements easily accessible during travel. Consider using a pill organizer for convenience.

Dining Out Tips:

Research Restaurants:

• Look up restaurant menus online in advance to identify options that are low in fat and suitable for your dietary needs.

• Consider calling ahead to discuss your dietary restrictions with the restaurant staff.

Order Wisely:

- Choose grilled, baked, or steamed dishes over fried or heavily sauced options.

- Ask for dressings and sauces on the side to control fat intake, or request alternatives like olive oil and vinegar.

Enzyme Replacement Therapy (ERT):

- Take enzyme supplements with every meal and snack as directed by your healthcare provider.

- Carry a travel-sized container of enzymes and a portable water bottle for convenience.

Portion Control:

- Opt for smaller portions or share larger dishes to avoid overloading your digestive system.

Be Prepared:

- Be prepared to educate restaurant staff about your dietary needs and the importance of enzyme supplements if needed.

- Have a list of foods that are easier for you to digest and ask about preparation methods if unsure.

Monitor Symptoms:

- Pay attention to any symptoms such as abdominal discomfort, bloating, or diarrhea, and adjust your food choices accordingly.

Enjoy the Experience:

- Despite dietary restrictions, focus on enjoying the dining experience and the company of others.

- Choose restaurants with a relaxed atmosphere where you can comfortably manage your meal.

By planning ahead, communicating your needs, and being proactive with enzyme replacement therapy, you can enjoy travel and dining out experiences while effectively managing Exocrine Pancreatic Insufficiency. Adapt these tips to suit your specific needs and consult with healthcare providers for personalized advice before traveling or dining out.

Lifestyle And Wellness Tips

Managing Exocrine Pancreatic Insufficiency (EPI) involves adopting a holistic approach to lifestyle and wellness. Here are some tips to support overall well-being for individuals with EPI:

1. Balanced Diet:

- **Nutrient-Dense Foods:** Focus on whole foods that are rich in nutrients such as lean proteins (chicken, turkey, fish), whole grains (quinoa, oats), fruits, and vegetables.
- **Low-Fat Choices:** Choose lean cuts of meat, skim or low-fat dairy products, and limit high-fat foods that may exacerbate symptoms.
- **Small, Frequent Meals:** Opt for smaller meals throughout the day to

aid digestion and nutrient absorption. Avoid large meals that can overwhelm the digestive system.

2. Enzyme Replacement Therapy (ERT):

- **Consistent Use:** Take pancreatic enzyme supplements with every meal and snack as prescribed by your healthcare provider.
- **Adjust Dosage:** Consult with your healthcare team to adjust enzyme dosages based on meal size, fat content, and individual response.

3. Hydration:

- **Drink Plenty of Water:** Stay hydrated throughout the day to support digestion and overall health. Aim for at least 8 glasses of water daily, adjusting based on individual needs.

4. Physical Activity:

- **Gentle Exercise:** Engage in regular physical activity such as walking, swimming, or yoga, as tolerated. Exercise can aid digestion and promote overall wellness.
- **Consult with Healthcare Provider:** Discuss appropriate exercise routines and any modifications needed based on individual health status and capabilities.

5. *Stress Management:*

- **Relaxation Techniques:** Practice stress-reducing activities such as deep breathing exercises, meditation, or mindfulness to promote relaxation and digestion.
- **Prioritize Rest:** Ensure adequate rest and sleep to support overall well-being and digestive health.

6. *Monitor Symptoms:*

- **Track Symptoms:** Keep a journal to monitor symptoms such as abdominal pain, bloating, diarrhea, or weight changes. This information can help identify triggers and guide treatment adjustments.
- **Regular Check-ups:** Attend regular appointments with your healthcare team for monitoring and adjustments to your treatment plan as needed.

7. *Social Support:*

- **Connect with Others:** Seek support from family, friends, or support groups who understand your condition and can provide encouragement and empathy.
- **Educate Loved Ones:** Help educate those close to you about EPI, its management, and dietary needs to foster understanding and support.

8. Stay Informed:

- **Educate Yourself:** Stay updated on new research, treatment options, and lifestyle strategies for managing EPI effectively.
- **Consult Healthcare Providers:** Ask questions and discuss any concerns with your healthcare team to ensure you have the most current information and guidance.

9. Adaptation and Flexibility:

- **Adjust as Needed:** Be flexible with your diet and lifestyle choices, adapting them based on your individual response to treatments and changes in health status.

By integrating these lifestyle and wellness tips into daily routines, individuals with Exocrine Pancreatic Insufficiency can optimize their health, manage symptoms effectively, and enhance their overall quality of life. Always consult with healthcare providers for personalized advice and guidance tailored to your specific needs and health goals.

CHAPTER ELEVEN
Monitoring Progress And Adjusting The Diet

Monitoring progress and adjusting the diet are crucial aspects of managing Exocrine Pancreatic Insufficiency (EPI) effectively. Here are some key steps and considerations for monitoring and adjusting the diet:

Monitoring Progress:

Symptom Tracking:

• Keep a detailed record of symptoms such as abdominal pain, bloating, diarrhea, constipation, weight changes, and overall digestive comfort.

- Note any patterns related to specific foods, meal sizes, or times of day.

Nutritional Status:

- Regularly assess nutritional status through discussions with healthcare providers, including monitoring weight, height (in children), BMI (Body Mass Index), and blood tests for vitamin and mineral levels.

- Check for signs of malnutrition or deficiencies, such as fatigue, weakness, or changes in skin, hair, or nails.

Enzyme Replacement Therapy (ERT) Effectiveness:

- Evaluate how well enzyme supplements are working by observing digestive symptoms after meals.

- Discuss any concerns or changes in symptoms with your healthcare team to adjust enzyme dosage or timing as needed.

Food Tolerance and Preferences:

- Note which foods are well-tolerated and which ones may trigger symptoms. Adjust the diet accordingly to minimize discomfort and optimize nutrient absorption.

- Consider preferences and challenges in meal planning to ensure dietary adherence and enjoyment.

Adjusting the Diet:

Consult with Healthcare Providers:

- Regularly review dietary strategies and progress with healthcare providers, including gastroenterologists and dietitians who specialize in managing EPI.

- Seek guidance on adjusting enzyme dosages, modifying meal plans, or addressing specific nutritional deficiencies.

Modify Fat Intake:

- Adjust the amount and type of fats in the diet based on tolerance levels. Choose healthier fats such as olive oil, avocados, and nuts, and limit saturated and trans fats.

- Use enzyme supplements with higher fat meals to aid digestion and absorption.

Balanced Nutrition:

• Ensure meals are balanced with adequate protein, carbohydrates, vitamins, and minerals to support overall health and well-being.

• Consider supplementation under the guidance of healthcare providers to address specific nutrient deficiencies if necessary.

Meal Planning Strategies:

• Plan meals that are nutrient-dense, easily digestible, and tailored to individual preferences and tolerances.

• Opt for smaller, more frequent meals throughout the day to ease digestion and manage symptoms.

Trial and Observation:

• Introduce new foods or variations in the diet gradually to observe their impact on symptoms and overall well-being.

• Keep a food diary to track responses to dietary changes and discuss findings with healthcare providers.

Educate and Empower:

• Educate yourself and others involved in meal preparation about dietary needs and strategies for managing EPI.

• Encourage open communication with family members, caregivers, and healthcare providers to optimize dietary adjustments and support.

Monitoring progress and adjusting the diet are ongoing processes in managing Exocrine Pancreatic Insufficiency. By staying proactive, documenting changes, consulting healthcare providers regularly, and making informed dietary choices, individuals can optimize their nutritional intake, manage symptoms effectively, and improve their overall quality of life. Each person's experience with EPI is unique, so personalized guidance from healthcare professionals is essential for tailored management strategies.

Conclusion

Managing Exocrine Pancreatic Insufficiency (EPI) requires a comprehensive approach that integrates dietary management, enzyme replacement therapy (ERT), lifestyle adjustments, and ongoing monitoring of symptoms and nutritional status. By focusing on these key aspects, individuals with EPI can effectively navigate the challenges associated with impaired pancreatic function and optimize their overall health and well-being.

Key strategies include:

- **Balanced Diet:** Emphasizing nutrient-dense foods, managing fat intake, and adjusting meal patterns to support digestion and nutrient absorption.
- **Enzyme Replacement Therapy (ERT):** Consistently using prescribed enzyme supplements with meals and

snacks to aid in the digestion of fats, proteins, and carbohydrates.

- **Lifestyle Modifications:** Incorporating regular physical activity, practicing stress management techniques, and prioritizing hydration and adequate rest.
- **Monitoring and Adjustment:** Tracking symptoms, nutritional status, and the effectiveness of ERT to make informed adjustments to the diet and treatment plan.
- **Collaboration with Healthcare Providers:** Working closely with gastroenterologists, dietitians, and other healthcare professionals to receive personalized guidance, address concerns, and optimize care.

Individuals with EPI can improve their quality of life, manage symptoms efficiently, and promote long-term health and wellness by applying these techniques and keeping open contact with healthcare practitioners. Achieving best outcomes and sustaining overall health requires personalized management techniques because each person's journey with EPI is unique.

THE END

www.ingramcontent.com/pod-product-compliance
Lightning Source LLC
Chambersburg PA
CBHW071826210526
45479CB00001B/16